Heart Health

An American Yoga Association Wellness Guide

Heart Health

An American Yoga Association
Wellness Guide

*The Complete Program for
New Strength and Vigor*

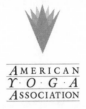

AMERICAN
Y·O·G·A
ASSOCIATION

Alice Christensen

The American Yoga Association

TWIN STREAMS
KENSINGTON PUBLISHING CORP.
http://www.kensingtonbooks.com

TWIN STREAMS BOOKS are published by

Kensington Publishing Corp.
850 Third Avenue
New York, NY 10022

ISBN 1-57566-662-6

Twin Streams and the TS logo are trademarks of Kensington Publishing Corp.

First Twin Streams Paperback Printing: May 2001
10 9 8 7 6 5 4 3 2 1

Printed in the United States of America

Photographs by Evelyn England, SAGE Productions
Hair and makeup by Estee Navarro and Ashley Kingston
Models: Patrick Benz, Pattie Cerar, Kent England, Linda Gajevski, Carole Guerin, Steve Honeyager, Steven Sanchez, Anne Wardwell, Ed Wardwell
Book design by Melody Oakes

READERS PLEASE NOTE: *The techniques and suggestions presented in this book are not intended to substitute for proper medical advice. Consult your physician before beginning any new exercise program. The American Yoga Association assumes no responsibility for injuries suffered while practicing these techniques. The American Yoga Association does not recommend Yoga exercise for pregnant or nursing women or for children under 16 years of age. If you are elderly or have any chronic or recurring conditions such as high blood pressure, neck or back pain, arthritis, heart disease, and other problems, please seek your physician's advice before practicing.*

Acknowledgments

I would like to thank the staff, students, and friends of the American Yoga Association for their help with this book, particularly Pattie Cerar and Carol Goodwin for general research assistance, Stephen Grant for nutritional research and writing, Linda Gajevski for development and production, and Patricia Rockwood for editorial assistance.

I would also like to thank the models for this book, including Steven Sanchez and Rodney Thompson, plus several students who have been with me for over 20 years: Patrick Benz, Pattie Cerar, Kent England, Linda Gajevski, Carole Guerin, Steve Honeyager, Anne Wardwell, and Ed Wardwell.

Table of Contents

Preface

I have never experienced heart problems myself, but I am familiar with the frightening aspects of a heart attack. I was present when my beloved teacher, Rama of Haridwar, suffered a massive coronary. It was the mid-1960s, and I had traveled to India with Rama for advanced study with him at his jungle retreat above Haridwar on the Ganges River. My initial visit of three months had been extended. I studied intensively, and traveled with Rama all over India as he lectured and taught. Much later I wrote a small book, called *Light of Yoga*, about those precious times; following is an excerpt that I thought might interest you, describing Rama's heart attack and the feelings that I experienced:

I was not prepared when Rama clutched his chest, turned deathly pale, and dropped to the floor one afternoon. We put him on his cot and tried desperately to revive him. It was a massive coronary. I saw all the signs and went running for my medicine kit for the drugs I had brought for an emergency. Why I had packed that particular medicine I will never know, but it was there. He was in terrible pain, pain so severe that he could barely speak. I held him in my arms, feeling in a crazy way that I could give him some of my own life and energy.

What can people do in such moments? He looked into my eyes with that look that has been with me and will be, the rest of my life. He said "The body invents a way to go. Alice, do not fear."

"You can't die. You can't die and leave me!" I argued, cried, and begged and finally in despair rocked back and forth like a madwoman on the edge of his cot. Inadequacy is the worst thing of all. One or two hours went by — I don't really know.

I sent our servant Balaji for Amar Singh — a man who worked as a servant in our camp during the day. Balaji said he had called him, but I knew he had not, so I went to his room and found that he had gone back to sleep on his cot. I went running off down the path of the compound screaming for Amar Singh all the way. I had driven a car from Delhi and I decided to try to get Rama to a hospital there, but I needed someone to show me the way. I did not speak the language, nor could I read the signs even if I were lucky enough to find the main road.

I found Amar Singh's hut in the dark. I knew he was an intelligent man and believed that between us, some way, we could communicate. I said, "Delhi, Delhi," and then "Rama, Rama," and clutching my heart tried to make him understand what had happened. He did, and we went at once to carry Rama to the car. Fixing a bed of sorts in the back, we started off in the night with Rama half conscious in the back.

I drove through the jungles all night, through the winding ways, with Amar Singh and I doing our best to see where to go. Finally we came to a town and stopped for water. I tried to wash Rama's face off a little and he revived slightly. He gasped, "Do you want me to live so much?"

I cried, "Rama, Rama, if you die my life is ended, don't die, you must not die."

He smiled a little and said very softly, "Then I will live for a little while yet."

I hurried back to the driver's seat and continued my mad rush in the night. After six hours of driving, we pulled into Delhi. (I still hold the record for driving time between Haridwar and Delhi.) Though I had never driven in the city before, I somehow managed to find Dr. Kelkar's house. I ran up the stairs and pounded on the door. Their little boy answered and was shocked to see me. Dr. Kelkar came running and then, of all things, I saw Rama get out of the car and stand up. I yelled wildly to carry him, that he had a heart attack, but Dr. Kelkar thought he had an excited woman on his hands. He totally ignored my warnings, paid no attention to me, and he and Rama walked up the stairs.

I was amazed when Rama said, "See that Amar Singh gets some tea."

They put him in a chair and called a doctor. She came at once and said that he must get to the hospital. We left again in the car and then waited at the hospital for two hours before anyone would do anything. I thought I would go out of my mind that day trying to get someone to pay attention to my pleas. How American I was; no one hurries like that in India.

The hospital was packed and busy. After many encounters and about six hours later, Rama was given a room and put to bed. The sheets on the bed were dirty; I found out later the previous patient had been a burned child. Under sedation, Rama began to muse pleasantly about the things that had happened in the last year while we were together. As he rambled on, I lay on the cot people had thoughtfully put there for me, and I remember giving him a glance to see if he was really breathing, and then I slept.

Next day the sun rose hot and hard. Outside the little room was a stone balcony. I walked out to see the few sheets and pillow cases being laid out on the grass to dry. Chickens walked around happily and I could see fire smoke starting as people got their morning meals ready. In India in those days, when a family member was taken to hospital, the whole family went along, setting up living quarters in the compound.

Rama was incoherent; the drugs evidently did their work well. About two or three days passed before I began to get the feeling of night and day. It was a matter of survival: one step at a time; one day at a time.

A boy came to clean the room. He had a pail of filthy water and started to wipe it around the place. I took the rag and water from him, changed it, and then started scrubbing the room myself. It suddenly felt good to be doing something — just anything. I looked around and found all the hospital authorities standing in distress watching me. A white woman just does not scrub floors, sweep, or clean there. I protested that in my country I did this every day. There was no shame in it; I wanted to do it.

Rama spoke quietly from his bed, "You are in India now." I did not clean the floors anymore; the boy they sent kept our floor shining clean for the peculiar taste of the American.

I lived there in that little hospital with Rama passing in and out of consciousness for about two weeks. I became rather strange. I spoke strangely, and lots of times I would catch myself talking to my sons and thinking that I was in some way hearing their words. Rama became better. His disciples brought food to us and other things that were needed.

I think I got pretty bad there for a while, because Dr. Kelkar took me home one night and told me he would stay with Rama for the night. He told me to get some rest and come back in the daytime. The next morning when I got a taxi just at dawn, the red sandstone of the India Gate was gleaming in the sun as we drove under it on the way to the hospital. Things were looking up. The doctors announced that Rama would live.

A letter came. I had been so anxious for my mail. It had been forwarded from Ram Kunj, our camp in the jungle, but it took a while to bring it to Delhi. I had looked so long for word from home. It seemed as though some word from there would comfort me so much. I opened the letter. It was from my husband, saying that he was leaving me. He was suing that I was an unfit mother and wanted a divorce immediately.

I felt a shock, and my whole world seemed to fall apart. Rama saw my shock. He grabbed the letter from my hand and, seeing what it said, told me that I must return home immediately. We stared at each other, neither one of us able to speak for a moment.

I told him that I could not go now and leave him like this. He said, "You must. Your children need you."

He arranged for his disciples to take me to the airline office, and they prepared an emergency ticket for me. A servant was sent to Ram Kunj for the few things that I wanted to take with me, and by the time he returned, my papers were in order. I stumbled through my last hours in India. When my clothes came I pulled out some slacks, long wrinkled from disuse, and pulled them on with a cotton shirt. I laid my gold-colored sari aside. Indian friends began to gather, and then I left for the hospital to say my last good-bye to my precious Guru.

I walked up the terrace steps still in the dream that had begun so long ago. The sweet night smell of India was there. I had packed my clothes with frangipani blossoms, and the odor clung to them. Rama mustered his strength and stood next to his bed. I protested, as I knew he was not supposed to move at all, but he said that I should remember him standing, not sick in bed. I had no tears left. We held each other closely and then I left.

Rama eventually recovered, and lived for several more years. I returned to India once more to see him, and he visited me in the United States as well.

Many people who read this story ask me how a Yoga master like Rama could have a heart problem. Yoga is supposed to be health-giving, they say. All I can say in response is that illness has many causes, not all of them related to physical and emotional conditioning; genetics, for instance, plays a big part. Yoga cannot promise perfect health and perfect cures; its promise — and this is a big one, when you think about it — is that it gives you the tools to bring yourself to the best physical and mental condition that you can to face the trials of your life. It has helped me tremendously and I hope it will help you, too.

Alice Christensen
Sarasota, Florida

Introduction

Most of us consider our heart to be the source of life, and the enjoyment of a perfectly working heart enhances life. Emotionally and physically we refer to our heart as the center of depth and joy that we can express and display in this world. In order to be able to do this, we need to protect and care for our heart in every possible way.

When we discover something is wrong with our heart, a deep depression often forms. This stops our ability to take steps to bring ourselves back to health using all the avenues open to us. One of the best ways I have found to assess any situation and work out what to do about it is to use a pencil-and-paper exercise.

Try this technique: Sit down in a quiet place, alone, away from distractions of any kind. Draw a line from top to bottom down the center of a piece of paper. You will be making two lists on the paper. On one side of the page, compose a list of what would give you completeness and happiness in this world — your deepest, most important desires and goals. Opposite each item, write what stands in the way of the fulfillment of that goal.

Make the list as long or short as you like. I have used this technique in my teaching, and sometimes the size of the lists is very revealing. One student made the list on a business card; another actually came in with a roll of wallpaper. Whatever type of paper you choose for your lists, make sure you have room to clearly see what you have written in both lists.

After you've made the two lists, read them over carefully, and think about two things:

1. How much time are you putting in to achieving the goals you have listed in the first column?

2. Looking at the second column, which of these obstacles depend upon a health problem? In other words, does your state of health stand in your way, keeping you from achieving your deepest desires and longings?

If you find that a health problem seems to be keeping you from achieving most of your goals, ask yourself if it is your attitude about your health, rather than a health problem itself, that holds you back. You may be surprised to find that a constant depression about the state of your health can convince you that (a) you cannot fight back, (b) you cannot help yourself, and therefore (c) you must give up and be sick the rest of your life. This does not have to be. A health problem is not a brick wall that keeps you from achieving your goals in life. For instance, many people who have angina or who are recovering from a heart attack believe that the exertion required by pastimes such as gardening, or social relationships, are too much for their heart. Talk it over with your doctor; most likely you will find that you can still enjoy most or all of the activities that give you pleasure and fulfillment; in fact, for most people, resuming activities that you enjoy can actually speed your recovery and reduce your risk of further heart injury.

Because our heart is the center of our being, when it is threatened it seems to affect everything else in life. Using a list like this will help you to avoid lumping everything in your life into one unapproachable pile and blaming the loss on your heart. You can sort out what you want to do and proceed, step by step, toward happy, balanced decisions. Take a hard look at what you want to do with your life and decide if you want to stand up and fight for it. Move on the specific obstacles that seem to stand in your way with a concentrated and formidable approach. Instead of giving in to depression, thinking, "Because I have a heart problem, all my hopes are unrealized," make a daily plan for yourself that addresses specific problems. Go through your list and decide what part of each day you will spend on efforts to achieve the desires you have listed, and you will find a very clear picture of what is most important to you and how to begin handling it.

Dealing with heart problems takes concentrated energy and time. You can help yourself greatly by adding simple physical exercises and simple breath techniques, such as are described in this book, to your daily schedule. Your diet needs to be carefully monitored, and this takes time. Many people at first dislike the lifestyle changes demanded by heart health programs and invent ways to disregard them. If you find yourself drifting into this pattern, use your list to remind yourself of what is most important to you in your life; this will reinforce your efforts toward necessary changes.

Change is always difficult, and motivation is important. Daily meditation, as a part of the program in this book, is the golden charm that will enable you to stick to your new regime. It will inspire you to fight back against this attack on your life. I think you will find desires and goals on your list that can be reached by creating a new outlook about yourself that will emerge from the practice of the routine described in this book. It will come quickly. You will notice a change in yourself in as little as a week if you follow the routine as it is presented. You can help heal an ailing heart and also help to prevent future heart problems. Take time to take care of your heart now and you will look forward to later years of strength and independence. The plan is easy to follow and will not frighten you with a future of unpleasant discipline.

The routine in this book will enable you to pull together all your options and bravely reach for recovery. If you have a heart problem that you are dealing with now, start slowly and enjoy a daily routine that is comfortable and pain-free, one that supports healing, allowing you to enjoy life. You can give your heart new support to continue its consistent operation throughout your life.

Although you will notice changes very quickly, this is not a two-week fix-up. Yoga practice is most helpful when it becomes part of a lifestyle that carries through your whole life. It becomes a pleasant habit that you will look forward to every day. In fact, once you begin, you will miss it if you don't practice. It is something that you will enjoy the rest of your life. It is time spent on yourself to enable you to be strong, clear-minded, and independent. Sometimes exercise routines become boring after a few weeks. You will not have that problem with this routine if you practice the Yoga exercises, breathing, and meditation altogether. If possible, do not split them up. Each day, before you begin your practice, visualize yourself and your heart as a strong, perfectly working unit. Your practice will become extremely pleasant. Most people who begin to practice Yoga never give it up.

I have been practicing Yoga for over 50 years now, and I must say that my heart is doing its job very well. I did have an experience, however, when my heart stopped, and I know what it feels like. It happened many years ago when I was living in India in the jungle above Haridwar with my teacher Rama. My youngest son, Eric — he was 18 at the time — was with me, and some other students as well. We were sitting on the small veranda outside our hut when suddenly my heart stopped. I fell forward on the floor in shock and pain, and started to lose consciousness. Eric lifted me to a cot, and Rama began to furiously work over me. He was terribly angry and kept yelling "This is mischief!" over and over. My heart finally started again, I came back to full consciousness, and things calmed down a bit. Rama told us that a man who lived in the deep grass near the river had done this to me and that he had made a bad mistake. This was true, it seems, because the hut where the fellow lived burned to a cinder soon after and he was never seen again. I was only 42 years old at the time, and I have never had any evidence of heart problems before or since.

I was fortunate that Rama was there to take care of me; not everyone has a Guru in the jungle to put things right. However, with this book, you now have powerful tools to help you take care of yourself. Be strong, be courageous. Life is all about fight. Yoga practice can teach you how to fight for your life; and your life is worth it.

Overview of This Book

You probably acquired this book for one of two reasons: either you believe you are at risk for heart disease and want to find out how to reduce that risk; or perhaps your doctor has diagnosed the beginning stages of heart disease and suggested that you make some lifestyle changes, including stress management, a low-fat diet, and more exercise. The techniques of Yoga are well known to help people cope with stress; you'll find out more about this important benefit in Chapter 2.

I have designed this book to be a program that you can follow easily on your own. However, everyone is different, and you may need to modify the program beyond the suggestions included in this book. I strongly suggest that you take this book to your personal physician and go over it together to make sure you are getting the most out of the program. This book cannot substitute for an ongoing relationship with the physician who is monitoring your heart condition, and you should never change your prescribed medication or regimen without consulting your physician.

I would like this book to give you a new way to approach a healthy heart, by learning how to move, breathe, eat, think, and feel, supplying proper attention to both your bodies, physical and emotional, that together are the basis for making you a whole person (see Chapter 2 for more about your two bodies).

Sometimes it helps to educate yourself about the situation you are facing. Chapter 1 outlines some basic information about heart health. Chapter 2 discusses in more detail the role of stress management in protecting your heart. Chapter 3 provides a full description of our Yoga program, including a detailed discussion of how the various components of the program — Yogic exercise, breathing techniques, meditation, fantasy, moderate exercise, and diet — work together to help you reach your goals.

Our Yoga program for heart health begins in Chapter 4, with complete instructions for the Yoga exercises, called asans, that I feel will be most helpful to you. Along with the exercise descriptions, I have included some additional material about the effects and benefits of each technique and some links to important nutritional advice. The program continues in the next three chapters: Chapter 5, with complete instruction in breathing techniques; Chapter 6, which teaches you how to relax completely and to meditate; and Chapter 7, which shows you how to use Fantasy to enhance your success.

This chapter teaches one of my favorite exercises: the "I Love You" Meditation Technique. This is a wonderfully effective technique that many of my students have used with great success to reduce depression and help them feel better about themselves. In Chapter 8, I introduce a way to incorporate moderate activity using walking, swimming, or stationary cycling in your Yoga program in order to improve the fitness of your heart and arteries.

Attention to diet and nutrition is essential to a healthy heart. A proper diet can improve your body's disease-fighting ability, repair tissues, and also help you lose weight. Chapters 9 and 10 show you how to modify your attitudes and tastes so that you can enjoy a healthy diet, with special attention to the components of your diet that will most help your heart and arteries.

Finally, a resource section lists support groups and organizations devoted to heart health, helpful Internet sites, and a reading list on exercise and nutrition. This section also discusses how to choose a qualified Yoga teacher and presents a complete list of the American Yoga Association's books and tapes on Yoga for further study.

Cautions and Hints

Consult Your Physician

I advise all my new students to consult their physicians before beginning Yoga practice, or any new exercise routine. Although the exercises and techniques in this book are meant for beginners, and are presented in a way that makes them easy to learn, it is a good idea to make sure that you have no underlying health problem that could cause complications. Your doctor can best tell you what movements you may need to avoid or modify in order to minimize your risk.

It is easy to modify the Yoga exercises in our program if you have been severely inactive, are convalescing, or suffer from other complications to your health such as arthritis. For many techniques, I've provided instructions for a seated version; many can even be done in bed. You can easily adapt most of the other techniques the same way. If you have any questions about modifying the exercises in this book, please write to me at the address printed in the Resources section. My book *Easy Does It Yoga* is an excellent supplemental resource, as it provides dozens of adapted Yoga exercises that can be done in a chair, bed, or pool. Our *Easy Does It Yoga Trainer's Guide* can help those of you who are helping someone else to recover.

Set Realistic Goals

Do not strain to do more than your body can do happily; this would violate the important Yogic ethic of Nonviolence, and if your body is feeling pain, you won't enjoy your practices. If you try to do too much at first, it may soon feel overwhelming. I would like you to enjoy this Yoga program, not look upon it as pain or drudgery. Set up a routine for yourself that you will enjoy.

Very few people have the time or desire to do a full Yogic exercise routine every day, and so I suggest starting with at least three of the exercises (in addition to the warm-ups) as your daily routine. Add more exercises whenever you wish, and gradually you will work into a fuller routine.

I would like to stress that your total daily commitment to our Yoga program, including Yoga exercise, breathing, meditation, fantasy, and brisk exercise, should not take more than one and one-half hours. This may seem like a major daily commitment, but you don't have to do the whole program all at once. For instance, try your 30 minutes of brisk exercise in the morning, a 20- to 30-minute routine of Yoga exercises, breathing, and meditation in the late afternoon or after work, and a fantasy technique just before bed to help you fall into normal sleep patterns.

Yoga seems very easy to do; however, it creates a powerful effect that is not always apparent when you are first starting out, and that is why I recommend only 20-30 minutes for the Yoga exercise, breathing, and meditation. Practicing for longer than this might upset your nervous system. You can practice in one continuous session or break your practice time into two 15-minute segments, morning and evening, although for best results I recommend that you try to practice the Yoga exercise, breathing, and meditation portions of the program consecutively.

Many times, in talking to people I meet all over the world, I am dismayed to hear them say, "We do three hours of meditation every day," or "We always start with an hour of breath exercises." When I hear statements such as these, I have to suspect that the instructor is incompetent, because this intensity of practice is very hard on the nervous system. If students can truly meditate 10 to 15 minutes, that puts them at the top of my class. It takes many years to slip into long meditation, and it can never be forced. It is very common for beginners to overdo simply because the routine helps them feel better. If you are new to exercise, you may feel so good initially that you "burn out" and quit. I suggest that you keep your daily routine short and interesting.

When to Practice Yoga Techniques

It does not matter what time of day you practice Yoga exercise, breathing, and meditation, although many people prefer early morning because their mind is not yet whirling with the day's activities. Whatever time of day you choose, the most important thing to remember is to practice a little every day. Even if you practice only three exercises, three Complete Breaths, and a few minutes of meditation, you will continue to build an underlying momentum of regular Yoga practice that will eventually make it as easy and natural to do as brushing your teeth every day. You will miss it if you don't do it.

Clothing, Equipment, Environment

Wear loose, warm, comfortable clothing for Yoga practice, appropriate for the season. Try to keep these clothes separate so you use them only for Yoga practice. Do not allow yourself to become either chilled or overheated. It's best to practice Yoga exercises barefoot, but be sure to put on a pair of socks before you lie down for meditation in order to keep your feet warm. Also, wrap your upper body in a shawl or sweater when you meditate, because your body temperature will drop, and a chill can upset your meditation period.

You do not need any special equipment to practice Yoga other than a large towel, blanket, or mat that you use only for Yoga practice, and one or two small, firm cushions for the seated breathing exercises, if you wish to sit on the floor for these techniques. Alternatively, any sturdy chair that won't tip over will suffice. You can also practice most breathing techniques, and many of the Yoga exercises, lying in bed.

Choose a place in your home that is quiet and free from drafts. If you have small children at home, try to fit your practice into the times when they are asleep or at school, so that your attention is not split from what you are doing. Turn your telephone ringer off so you will not be startled by loud noise, and be sure you will not be disturbed by pets.

Scheduling

Although the different parts of your Yoga routine — exercise, breathing, and meditation — will work best if done consecutively, sometimes your schedule or family obligations may not allow that much time all at once. In that case, it's fine to split up your routine, although I suggest that you keep breathing and meditation together. For instance, you could practice breathing and meditation in the morning and your exercise routine in the evening. Just be sure to practice a little every day without fail.

Food, Caffeine, Alcohol, Medication

Wait about two hours after eating a large meal so that you are not practicing Yoga exercises on a full stomach. However, a light snack or beverage before exercising will not hurt. Try to avoid practicing immediately after ingesting caffeine, because caffeine will upset your meditation practice. Never practice Yoga under the influence of alcohol or street drugs. If you are taking any prescription medications that make you drowsy, wait until the effects have lessened before starting your Yoga routine.

Women's Issues

Women should not practice Yoga exercises during the heavy days of their menstrual cycle. The pressure of Yoga exercises on the internal organs may disrupt the natural hormonal changes of the body. Use the extra time for meditation, or spend a little more time on your walking exercises (see Chapter 8).

If you are pregnant or nursing, we do not recommend that you practice all the Yoga exercises because the changes in your body caused by the compression on internal organs may affect your child. A special routine for pregnant and nursing mothers is provided in two of our beginning books, *The American Yoga Association Beginner's Manual* and *20-Minute Yoga Workouts* (see Resources). However, we do suggest that you continue your Complete Breath and meditation practice every day, as well as the Walking Contemplation exercise outlined in Chapter 8. I find that the use of Fantasy is very helpful for a comfortable pregnancy.

Supplemental Instruction

Yoga is best practiced alone, and for this reason I have designed this book to be your personal Yoga teacher. If you decide that you would prefer to supplement the course of study in this book with support from a local Yoga class, see the Resources for a discussion of some qualities to look for in a good Yoga teacher and a few suggestions about where to start looking. Also see the Resources for our excellent videotape that leads you through a basic 30-minute Yoga class of exercise, breathing, and meditation such as I teach for the American Yoga Association.

I hope that you enjoy this program of Yoga for heart health. If you have any questions about what you are doing, please feel free to write to me at the address given in the Resources.

Chapter 1

Some Facts About Heart Health

Your cardiovascular system, which includes miles of arteries and blood vessels as well as the heart itself, is responsible for delivering oxygen and nutrients to your body's organs and removing waste products from the over 300 trillion cells in your body. The heart never rests, except for a split second between beats.

The heart and its arteries can become diseased or weakened through lack of exercise, a diet high in cholesterol and certain fats, smoking, and some genetic factors. Nearly 10% of the population (about 20 million people) have some form of heart disease, and 25% (63 million) have hypertension. About 30% of those with heart disease suffer limitations in their usual activities due to the disease. Women usually develop far fewer heart problems than men until they reach menopause and lose the protective properties of estrogen.

First described in the ancient world, coronary heart disease (CHD) was very rare until the advent of industrialization. Angina (severe pain in chest, shoulders, or other areas, associated with insufficient blood supply to the heart) was considered rare well into the 20th century, but an epidemic of it seized industrialized nations following the proliferation of the automobile and the prosperity and overly rich diet of our current times. CHD is the leading cause of death in the United States and accounts for one-fourth of all deaths over the age of 35. Most hospitalizations are due to CHD. CHD often goes unrecognized until it is too late; more than half of people who die from a heart attack have had no previous symptoms of heart disease.

The good news, however, is that heart disease is almost entirely preventable with lifestyle changes such as eating a low-cholesterol and low-fat diet, getting more exercise, and improving stress responses with Yoga techniques. Quitting smoking, of course, is absolutely imperative. The number of people with heart disease has been slowly declining since the mid-1960s, and the death rate from cardiovascular disease has actually declined 50% over the past 25 years — a testament to improved medical care as well as increased awareness of preventive lifestyle factors. More and more people seem to be willing to take responsibility for their own health.

What Is Heart Disease?

A healthy heart is one that receives a constant supply of blood from the coronary arteries that surround it. When these arteries start to become blocked, the potential for damage to the heart increases as its blood supply is reduced. A person is said to have coronary heart disease (CHD) or "atherosclerosis" when the coronary arteries are blocked to some degree (from "atheroma," meaning accumulation, and "sclerosis," meaning hardening). In simple terms, fatty deposits in the artery walls develop into hardened plaques that, over time, can considerably reduce blood flow. A leading cause of heart attacks is when blood flow to the heart is partially or completely stopped, often due to a blood clot. Clots usually form in the region of plaques, because either (a) the surfaces of plaques, unlike walls of healthy arteries, lack the protective substances that keep blood platelets from sticking to it and forming clots; or (b) plaques become brittle as they age and grow; they can rupture into the artery, triggering a natural wound-healing response that clots the blood.

Plaques can form in arteries throughout the body, but in this book we will be talking about only those arteries that surround and feed the heart, the coronary arteries. The name "coronary" refers to the crown or "corona" shape of the collection of arteries that feed the heart. The coronary arteries carry the life blood of the heart itself; they have nothing to do with the vessels involved in the heart's pumping action. With time, arterial plaques can harden, stiffening the arteries and further interfering with blood flow (thus the common term "hardening of the arteries").

Sometimes these blockages cause pain in the chest, shoulders, or other areas, called angina, that is often the only signal that the heart is in danger; however, as mentioned earlier, many times a person remains symptom-free until the blockages are so severe that they starve the heart and cause it to fail completely. Angina often appears after exertion, heavy meals, or stress, because during those times the heart has to work harder, and has an increased need for oxygen from the blood. Arteries that are partially blocked cannot let enough blood through to adequately nourish the heart in times of heavy demand.

The Cholesterol Story

The primary culprit in the formation of plaques is cholesterol, a soft, waxy substance that is present in all parts of the body, including the nervous system, endocrine glands, skin, muscles, liver, intestines, and heart. Cholesterol is necessary for cell structure, hormone production, and other uses. The body makes about 70% of its cholesterol; the remainder comes from dietary sources. Egg yolks (not whites) and organ meats are the highest dietary sources; other meat and dairy products (except nonfat) all contribute dietary cholesterol. Plant foods — fruit, vegetables, grains, nuts, and seeds — contain no cholesterol.

Our blood contains two different kinds of "lipids," or fats: fatty acids, mostly in the form of triglycerides, and cholesterol. There are two main types of cholesterol: HDL, or high-density lipoprotein, known as the "good" cholesterol, because it helps to remove waste cholesterol from the bloodstream; and LDL, or low-density lipoprotein, known as "bad" cholesterol, because it carries normal and excess amounts of cholesterol into the arteries. If cholesterol is not used by the cells it can combine with oxygen and lead to the formation of plaques. HDL can be increased by stopping smoking, achieving a reasonable weight, and exercising regularly. LDL can be reduced by eating a diet low in cholesterol and saturated fats.

Lipoproteins are like special transport vehicles that carry cholesterol to and from the cells and the liver. They are particles with a "shell" of protein, lecithin, and cholesterol that surrounds a "core" that is essentially an oily droplet of more cholesterol and fats. LDL particles transport cholesterol from the liver to the cells, which have special receptors that trap the cholesterol, pulling about 70% of it out of the bloodstream. HDL particles act as the bloodstream's "trash collector," picking up cholesterol that the cells throw off as they die and as they grow, and carrying it back to the liver to be excreted. Scientists now believe that we each have a finite number of LDL receptors, and thus a fixed capacity to absorb cholesterol, which varies from person to person.

Overwhelming your cells' LDL receptors by overfeeding with saturated fat and cholesterol can lead to the chronically high levels of LDL in the blood that spell trouble for your heart and arteries. There are many other factors that influence the body's ability to handle cholesterol, not all of them fully understood. This is why you will often have the frustrating experience of hearing some people boast about how, even though they have eaten eggs and bacon for breakfast their entire lives, they still have a healthy heart and a low cholesterol count!

If you have any symptoms of CHD, such as angina, or if you have two or more of the known risk factors — over 45 years of age (men) or 54 (women), overweight, diabetes, a history of smoking, or one or more relatives with premature heart disease — your doctor has probably advised you to have your cholesterol levels measured regularly. Cholesterol levels vary from day to day, so experts advise people to be tested more than once and average the results. Usually the results show five different values, four of which are expressed as concentrations in the blood (mg/dL, or milligrams per deciliter): total cholesterol, LDL, HDL, and triglycerides (see sidebar). The fifth number is the ratio of total cholesterol to HDL, a very important value for determining risk (see Chapter 10, p. 204). Levels in healthy people are generally under 200 total cholesterol, under 130 LDL, and over 35 HDL. The optimal total-to-HDL ratio is 4.0 or under. There is no agreed-upon acceptable value for triglycerides: expert opinions

What are Triglycerides?

Most fats in food, in our blood, and in storage in the body's fat cells are in the form of triglycerides and, with cholesterol, form the bulk of blood plasma fats in circulation. Triglycerides are the molecules into which all dietary fatty acids, whether unsaturated or saturated, are assembled for circulation and storage in the body, and their composition varies as our diet changes. When we eat mostly unsaturated fats, our triglycerides have a higher percentage of those unsaturated fats, and so forth. High triglycerides, like high saturated fats, seem to cause high cholesterol, but a diet low in saturated fat does not always reduce triglycerides. Experts do not know exactly what causes high triglycerides; it seems that underlying conditions such as diabetes or overweight may be at fault. If regular measurements of your triglyceride level tend to be high, your doctor will certainly want to find out why.

vary from under 250 to under 200. Please remember, however, that everyone is different, and your doctor is the only one who can interpret your results accurately. Depending upon the combination of these values, which vary from person to person, your doctor may advise you to be retested every two to five years and may start you on lifestyle changes such as dietary therapy, prescribe cholesterol-lowering drugs, or a combination.

Many people confuse "fats" with cholesterol; they are not the same, although they are related. A diet high in saturated fats can increase the level of cholesterol in the blood. Saturated fats are found primarily in animal products — meat and butterfat — as well as in a few vegetable fats such as palm and coconut oils and cocoa butter. Other factors, such as diabetes, kidney failure, low

HDL, and overweight, can also increase the level of fats in the bloodstream.

Fats that are not saturated are not harmful (in reasonable quantities) and can be beneficial, even helping to lower LDL and raise levels of HDL in the blood. If your cholesterol and triglyceride levels are dangerously high, you will probably be advised to reduce dietary fats to a maximum of 30% of total calories, with the bulk coming from vegetable sources to reduce saturated fats. If you simply need to cut down on your saturated fat intake, it is a good idea to substitute the more beneficial plant-based unsaturated fats for cholesterol and saturated fats. See Chapter 9 for a more thorough discussion of the different types of fats and the foods that contain them.

Here is an easy way to tell which fat is which: Saturated fats (also called hydrogenated fats) are almost always solid at room temperature: examples are butter, lard, shortening, and some margarines; many baked goods are made with other common saturated fats such as palm oil, coconut oil, and cocoa butter. "Partially hydrogenated" oils, which you will see as an ingredient in many baked and fried foods and many margarines, should be considered almost as harmful as saturated fats. They are widely used for frying and baking by restaurants and food manufacturers because they do not become rancid as quickly as most healthier oils and so they are considerably cheaper. "Trans" fatty acids are much in the news these days; trans fats are produced by hydrogenation, and are just as dangerous for your heart and arteries. Manufacturers are not yet required to list the amount of trans fat in a product label, but if you avoid saturated and partially or fully hydrogenated oils, you will avoid most trans fats.

Unsaturated fats, whether "monounsaturated" or "polyunsaturated," are usually liquid at room temperature. Some examples of monounsaturated fats are olive, peanut, and canola oils. Some examples of polyunsaturated fats are corn, safflower, sesame, and soy oils, and nuts and seeds. In Chapter 9, I will discuss more about how to modify your dietary intake of fats.

Other Risk Factors for CHD

Many risk factors contribute to the amount of fatty substances in the blood and the tendency of plaques to form. Some of these, such as smoking, high blood pressure, obesity, and dietary fat intake, we can do something about; others, such as age, gender, body type, and heredity, we cannot, though we can minimize the negative effects through positive lifestyle changes. Let's look at each of these risk factors in more detail:

Smoking

Cigarette smoking damages the artery lining, constricts arteries, increases clotting, and increases the heart's oxygen requirements. Quitting smoking reduces risk about 50% the first year; often your HDL levels will rise about 10% in the first month alone. The risk reduces almost to the level of nonsmokers during the next one to ten years. You may not find it so difficult to quit if you fully understand its importance. If you do have trouble, nicotine gum and patches, group support, or even hypnosis might do the trick. If you are trying to quit, I think you will find that regular Yoga practice will help greatly. Smoking, like other addictions, often has its roots in a poor relationship with the emotional body (see Chapter 2). As you improve general health and well-being, strengthen your nervous system, and learn to listen to the intuitive voice of your emotional body and follow its suggestions, you will find that you will crave nicotine less and less. It's almost as if the addiction gives you up rather than the other way around, allowing you to quit in a way that is nonviolent toward both your bodies.

Hypertension

High blood pressure, untreated, increases the damage to arteries done by high cholesterol, cigarette smoking, and diabetes. The greater the systolic (higher) number, the greater the risk for CHD. Some drugs that are prescribed for high blood pressure actually increase blood sugar, cholesterol, and fats, increasing the risk for CHD. Balancing all these factors can be managed only by your physician, who will probably recommend weight reduction, decreased sodium intake, and regular exercise in addition to or instead of drug therapy for hypertension. A regular Yoga program has been proven to greatly improve blood pressure, reducing dependence upon drugs; however, you should never stop taking any medication without consulting your doctor.

Overweight

Nearly half the population of the United States is at least mildly overweight. Moderate to severe obesity (weight greater than 30% to 40% above average) increases the risk of CHD dramatically, especially in the young. The distribution of body fat also seems to affect risk: those with predominantly abdominal fat (most men) are at greater risk than those with fat lower on the hips and thighs (most women).

Even moderate weight reductions of as little as 10% can have a marked influence on risk, though it may take at least a 20% reduction to improve angina. A common condition in obesity is sleep apnea, in which the person stops breathing for a few moments during sleep. When combined with CHD, this condition can cause dangerous irregularities in the heart's rhythm.

If you are overweight and seriously follow a diet low in fat and cholesterol, you will have no trouble losing weight as long as you don't substitute refined carbohydrates, such as white flour and sugar, and alcohol for the calories that you are cutting out in fat. Consult your physician or a registered dietician for help if you are moderately to severely overweight; if you are mildly overweight, our *Weight Management* book in this Wellness Guide series (see Resources) can offer some helpful suggestions for how to start losing weight safely. Chapter 10 also includes a few tips on how to begin.

Other Factors that Affect Cholesterol

Alcohol has variable effects: it can raise cholesterol and triglyceride levels, but it can also increase HDL. Large amounts of coffee (nine or more cups daily) elevate cholesterol levels. Higher levels of homocysteine, associated with low levels of vitamin B-12, folic acid, and B-6, may raise the risk of CHD. People with high stored iron levels combined with high LDL concentrations have increased risk of CHD.

On the positive side, nuts, especially walnuts (in moderation, of course) provide a heart-healthy source for antioxidants, flavonoids, and unsaturated fats. Dietary fiber also helps reduce cholesterol.

Diabetes

Diabetes manifests in two ways: Type I, glucose intolerance, means that the body produces little or no insulin, the hormone whose job it is to pull glucose (sugar) out of the bloodstream to be used by the cells. Type 2, insulin resistance, means that the body may have plenty of insulin but somehow the insulin is unable to link up with the cells so they can receive the glucose. If you have either type of diabetes, you are likely to have other risk factors for heart disease such as hypertension, obesity, and low HDL. Women who are diabetic do not benefit from the protective effect of estrogen, as nondiabetics do. High levels of blood glucose, caused by poor management of diabetes, can damage blood vessels over time. Diabetics — particularly those under 30 — also seem to have a higher incidence of calcium deposits in the blood vessels, a precursor to the formation of plaques. Diabetes and heart disease require most of the same lifestyle changes for successful management. Some experts believe that successful management of diabetes may substantially reduce the risk of heart disease.

"Guilt by Association"

You may have noticed that the above risk factors seem to be interrelated. If you have one or more of these conditions, you are at risk for some or all of the others. Which one manifests first is probably a function of your lifestyle and your heredity, or simply which is diagnosed first by your physician. What you must not forget, however, is that no matter how dire these risks sound, you can do something about each one of them. By changing your lifestyle now, you can reduce or eliminate your risk for heart disease.

As I mentioned previously, there are also risk factors that you cannot alter, such as age, gender, and family history. Professionals agree, however, that no matter how many risk factors you start with, no lifestyle changes will be wasted in helping you achieve better health. Here, then, are the primary risk factors for coronary heart disease:

- Age (men over 44, women over 54)
- Gender (men tend to have higher LDL and lower HDL than women)
- Family history (a close relative with premature heart disease)
- Diabetes
- Uncontrolled hypertension
- Smoking
- Overweight

If you have two or more of the above risk factors, start now to make the lifestyle changes that will reduce your risk. Artery blockages can start in people as young as age 25; in fact, some studies have found alarmingly high cholesterol levels in teenagers. Without attention to diet and other lifestyle changes, blockages slowly increase with age.

Estrogen Loss

Estrogen seems to help nondiabetic women avoid heart disease until they reach menopause, when estrogen levels naturally decline. Women who choose hormone replacement therapy (HRT) can reduce this risk, as well as protect themselves against osteoporosis, or bone loss, but HRT carries its own risks for breast and uterine cancer. You and your doctor must weigh the options and decide what is best for you.

To summarize, you can prevent most incidence of heart disease by doing the following:

- Regulate estrogen level (if you are a postmenopausal woman)
- Achieve and maintain a reasonable weight
- Stop smoking
- Reduce blood pressure (if you are hypertensive)
- Control blood sugar (if you are diabetic)
- Reduce dietary fats and cholesterol, eat a nutritious whole-foods diet, and add specific heart-healthy nutrients such as fiber, antioxidants, and high linoleic acid oils (see Chapters 9 and 10)
- Reduce or modify negative stress responses (see Chapter 2)
- Increase activity level (see Chapter 8)

Treatment Options

After all is said and done, it comes down to changing the way we eat, exercise, and react to everyday stress. Low-fat and low-cholesterol diets almost always reduce high levels of total and LDL cholesterol enough to significantly reduce CHD risk. An ever-growing field of research is also generating evidence that for those who are motivated to undertake extremely low-fat diets, even existing plaques in the arteries can be reduced in size and new ones prevented from forming — essentially reversing heart disease (see page 29). When you combine an improved diet with exercise that strengthens the heart muscle and improves overall fitness, and stress management skills that improve our response to stress, such as the program outlined in this book, you can make real progress toward healing damaged heart arteries. If you already have CHD, you have the opportunity for a whole new life free of angina pain and disability.

The first treatment of choice is dietary therapy. If you are unable to follow a careful diet and exercise program, or if you are one of the rare people for whom these measures are insufficient to reduce total cholesterol and LDL to safer levels, a number of drugs are now available to lower blood cholesterol levels. Some of the most common drug treatments, often used in combination, are described below:

1. Aspirin and other anticoagulants work to reduce the blood's ability to clot; clots can clog an artery that is already narrowed by plaques, resulting in even less flow to the heart.

2. Bile acid sequestrants, for example, Questran and Colestid, reduce LDL by trapping ("sequestering") cholesterol secreted by the liver as bile in the intestine.

3. Niacin, a common B vitamin, reduces LDL and raises HDL. However, up to one-third of patients do not tolerate large doses well due to significant side effects, and super-high doses can be toxic to the liver.

4. Enzyme inhibitors (statins), for example, Lipitor, Mevacor, Pravacol, and Zocor, lower cholesterol by inhibiting a critical

enzyme needed to synthesize cholesterol in the liver. As liver cholesterol drops, more is withdrawn from the bloodstream, lowering LDL by as much as 20-40%.

It is important to follow your physician's instructions completely when taking medication. Do not change or stop taking your medication without consulting your doctor.

Some fatty acids found naturally in foods such as flaxseed oil and fish oils have proved to be beneficial for lowering cholesterol levels as part of a low-fat, low-cholesterol diet. Substances called antioxidants also seem to protect our bodies from CHD. Read more about these heart-healthy nutrients as part of a complete cholesterol-lowering diet program in Chapter 9.

If the arteries are narrowed to a dangerous extent, surgery may be called for. Some now-routine procedures are bypass surgery, balloon angioplasty, and thrombolytic infusions for acute heart attacks. However, don't forget that surgery simply relieves the symptom of angina; it does nothing to change the underlying disease process, which still progresses in the remaining and repaired arteries. This is why, without lifestyle changes, many people need a repeat bypass operation in just a few years. The benefits of angioplasty are even shorter-lived. The only way to stop or reverse the artery-clogging process is to reduce cholesterol levels in the bloodstream through diet, exercise, other lifestyle changes and, if necessary, drug therapy.

Exercise by itself cannot either prevent or cure cardiac illness, but it can strengthen the heart muscle in the same way that it strengthens muscles throughout the body: by increasing its oxygen consumption. To achieve this effect, you have to work the heart muscle to 60% to 75% of its capacity, a measure called "target heart rate." See Chapter 8 for more about how to measure heart rate and structure your exercise sessions. Yoga exercise has a beneficial effect on the heart muscle; through localized pressure and carefully designed stretches, Yoga exercises, called asans, improve circulation throughout the body and strengthen and relax the sympathetic and autonomic nervous systems.

Lifestyle Changes Work

Over the past decade, several cardiologists have conducted research studies on the effects of drastic lifestyle change on patients with CHD. Dean Ornish, MD, is probably the most well known; his book *Dr. Dean Ornish's Program for Reversing Heart Disease* brought his methods to the attention of a wide public. His research in California, as well as that of Caldwell Esselstyn, MD, at the Cleveland Clinic and a group of German researchers, has also been described in professional journals such as *The Journal of the American Medical Association* and *The American Journal of Cardiology*. Dr. Ornish's program is the only one to incorporate regular Yoga practice, which he refers to as stress management training, as well as aerobic exercise and group support as integral parts of the intervention program. Other studies concentrated primarily on plant-based, very-low-fat diets and moderate exercise.

The goal of Dr. Ornish's initial research program was to see if an intensive lifestyle-changing program could reduce blockages in the coronary arteries and thus improve blood flow. Participants in the experimental group received no drugs, instead relying on a very low-fat, whole-foods vegetarian diet, aerobic exercise, stress management training, and group psychological support. The control group made more moderate changes in their lifestyle as directed by their physician according to standards of usual care.

The study followed participants for five years. On average, the experimental group showed continued improvement (regression of blockages) over the entire five years, while the control group actually regressed over the same period, despite receiving cholesterol-lowering drugs and even, in some cases, bypass surgery. The experimental group reduced LDL cholesterol by 40% at the end of one year and sustained a level of 20% reduction after five years, results comparable to drug treatment.

A second, larger study was undertaken with the goal of training teams across the country to motivate cardiac patients to follow similar intensive lifestyle changes, and to determine if this strategy was more cost-effective than revascularization (referring to either bypass surgery or angioplasty); in other words, to find out if such costly procedures could be safely prevented through lifestyle changes. Remarkably, the study was partially funded by about 40 insurance companies.

Teams of health professionals at eight sites around the country were trained in the program. A total of 333 patients completed the three-year program: 194 in the experimental group, all of whom were candidates for angioplasty or bypass surgery, and 139 in the control group, all of whom had just undergone one of those procedures.

Participants in the experimental group followed the same lifestyle program as in the original study, and results were similar. Of the 194 patients in the experimental group, 150 were able to avoid surgery during the three years of the program. After three years, LDL had dropped from 123 to 102, total cholesterol dropped from 202 to 183, triglyceride levels fell from 230 to 201, and HDL increased from 37 to 42. Participants lost an average of seven pounds, with other beneficial changes in percent body fat and exercise capacity.

The authors stress that comprehensive lifestyle changes are not for everyone; the attitude of someone willing to completely change his or her lifestyle is often quite different from someone who chooses surgery. Lifestyle changes require commitment, discipline, and a willingness to assume responsibility for one's own health. In contrast, patients who choose surgery tend to want the physician to "fix" them. Comprehensive lifestyle changes usually result in a rapid decrease in angina and other symptoms within weeks; these immediate benefits are highly rewarding and motivating. It also appears that although the risks of surgery increase with age, the benefits of changing your lifestyle are not age related. Older patients benefited as much as younger ones in the study because the only factor that mattered was the degree of adherence to the program.

Since the results of that most recent study were published, Dr. Ornish's training program has been expanded to 15 sites. Other independent studies have confirmed that lifestyle changes can work to both prevent and reverse heart disease.

Whether you and your doctor choose drug therapy, lifestyle changes, or a combination of the two, you will likely be following that program for the rest of your life. If your doctor approves, why not choose lifestyle change and reap the many extra benefits?

We have in our own hands the ability to prevent most incidences of heart disease: we can lower blood fats with diet and/or drugs, stop smoking, maintain a reasonable weight, normalize blood pressure through diet and exercise, learn to reduce negative stress responses, and add plenty of heart-healthy nutrients to our diet. This is the essence of our Yoga program for a healthy heart.

Chapter 2

Stress Management and Your Heart

It seems as if every health magazine on the newsstands contains an article about how to either reduce the stress in your life or help you manage it more effectively. There is no denying that stress is a constant in life. What you may not realize is that the changes in your physical body and the continual strain on your emotional body caused by prolonged stress reactions can be a major risk factor in coronary heart disease.

Your Two Bodies

In Yoga, we recognize that every individual actually has two bodies: the physical body that can be seen and touched, and an inner body that I call the "emotional/spiritual" body. I use these terms because the inner body is where your feelings, intuition, and self-awareness reside. Successful change in the physical body, by which I mean the ability to handle stress in the least self-harmful manner possible, calls upon the support of the inner emotional/spiritual body. Learning new stress-coping skills

The Risk of Depression

Several studies have looked at the connection between depression and heart problems, finding that people who report depressive symptoms are much more likely to develop heart disease than those who don't — especially among the elderly. Depression is very common in the elderly, though fewer than one percent get proper treatment. Many experts view depression as an extreme and prolonged response to stress. Depression may predict heart problems for several reasons: (a) People who feel depressed are less likely to exercise or stick with other preventive lifestyle changes such as eating a healthy diet, and they are more likely to medicate themselves with nicotine, alcohol, or drugs; (b) depression increases mental stress, which in turn can increase plaque formation and blockages in the vessels; and (c) it is possible that depression increases production of free radicals and fatty acids, which can damage the lining of blood vessels. The next research step will be to determine whether treating people for depression can stop or slow down the progression of heart disease.

is essentially a process of changing the way you respond to stress both physically and emotionally, and change is never possible without a balance between the two bodies. The word Yoga is from the Sanskrit "yug," meaning to join or bring together. The practice of Yoga is then the process of bringing the two bodies together in balance. In other words, you develop a harmonious relationship with yourself.

In most people, the two bodies are constantly at odds with each other, simply because they have never learned to work together. For instance, your physical body may be feeling fearful about angina pain, or dread at facing the discipline and "deprivation" of lifestyle changes; it does not realize that the inner body can be a source of great reassurance and help, because it speaks from a depth of intuitive understanding unknown to the physical body. When dealing with the effects of heart problems felt by your physical body, it will help you greatly to realize that you can call on your inner emotional body for support. Imagine having an invisible Siamese twin at your side; once you recognize and appreciate its contribution to your total health, it offers constant support. Practicing a regular Yoga routine will help you to find balance, compassion, and oneness with both your bodies, giving you the strength to make positive changes that help you enjoy life more.

If both bodies are not addressed, efforts to change usually fail. The lifestyle changes go on for a little while, but after some time the inner body tires of the game and comes back full force to return the outer physical body to its previous state, very much like a fussy housekeeper who, every time someone moves a piece of furniture, hastily returns it to its previous position for her personal satisfaction.

It seems paradoxical that a part of you would wish to return to a state of pain or discomfort, yet we often resist change because it represents the unknown; on the other hand, staying as we are, even if it means being in pain, is familiar and seems less stressful. This becomes more and more true the longer the painful condition persists. You may remember the old allegory about the man who had lived in a cave his entire life and had never seen the sun. When he was brought out into the sunshine for the first time, he ran back into the darkness that was familiar.

If you truly want to change the way you feel, you must call a board meeting with yourself where both bodies are in attendance. Both bodies must be consulted for a happy agreement to the change. Yoga techniques help to transform what is often a battlefield between the two parts of ourselves into a peaceful ground of understanding and appreciation of the needs of both bodies.

It may be a difficult meeting at first, because the two bodies are not used to talking with each other. The physical body has no idea of the power of the emotional body; it marches in demanding change as if it had all the answers. The emotional body listens and observes the physical's whining demands with lofty detachment. Each side maintains its separateness while the meeting goes on, and so nothing comes to agreement.

Try to imagine this scene played over and over again a hundred times as we try to change our lives. How many times have you tried to force your physical self to do something and failed? I have observed people doing terrible things to their bodies in order to force a result. The emotional/spiritual body usually resents it so much that after a while it demands drugs, alcohol, or other destructive escapes to mask the upset.

Yoga philosophy believes that complete power lies in the inner body, the emotional/spiritual body, which never changes or dies. The fragile physical body, which is born and dies, actually only functions because of the strength and compassion of the inner body. If the two bodies can be encouraged to work together, the balance that is achieved makes any change possible.

The whole system of Yoga was designed exactly for this purpose: to bring both parts of yourself together to work in harmony. When this happens, the inner battles with yourself

Listening to the Inner Body

One of my students wrote me to describe how she practiced listening for the voice of her inner body: "I had to meet a new client for my video-memoirs business: a mother-daughter team. Before I met them, I sat down, quieted myself, and turned inward to my spiritual body. I visualized the name of the mother on my mental screen. I got the impression of a strong, resilient, and resourceful woman. Then I saw her dancing on stage, though I wasn't sure what that meant. I did the same with the daughter and got the idea that she loved her mother very much. I saw her with wings like an angel, which puzzled me.

When I met the two women, I found out that the mother was from a Russian village that suffered many Cossack attacks. As a child, she had walked from Russia to France with her mother and brother. They hid during the day and walked at night for a year. She loved performers and loved being in front of my video camera. The daughter expressed her love for her mother, and her mother called her 'my angel.' Within minutes of meeting them, I realized my inner body had given me correct information and we were on the same wavelength instantaneously.

I also practiced this technique when my boyfriend and I were deciding whether to purchase the house we were renting. We both had mixed feelings about it. When I quieted myself, turned inward, and pictured the address, I got a very clear 'No.' My boyfriend had the same experience. Needless to say, we decided not to buy the house.

transform into clear, bright insights of intuition and practicality. The expressions of the inner body's presence and power then are able to show in balancing all the activities of your life.

If you give the unseen inner body expression, it will stop all resistance. It wants expression, and that can be done happily only if the outer physical body welcomes it. This friendly attitude developing in yourself then allows the strength of both bodies to come together in force, supporting all you want to do.

Stress and Your Two Bodies

I would like you to look upon the Yoga routine that you learn in this book not as a tranquilizer to calm your physical body, but as a way to communicate with both your bodies in a way that reduces the stress they both carry.

A stress response in the physical body is usually considered positive, because it prepares the body to adapt to new challenges, to be aware of danger or opportunity, or to help us survive in other ways. The body is equipped to respond to stress appropriately and then to recover in a fairly short time. It is when the stress response is sustained and pervasive — and when the emotional body is not acknowledged — that stress then poses a danger to health.

The coronary arteries are quite sensitive to stress, especially when they start to become clogged. The lining of the arteries produces a substance that helps to relax and dilate the arteries, allowing more blood to flow to the heart. When the lining becomes damaged by the plaques and thickening of atherosclerosis, less of this substance is produced, and so the arteries constrict more and relax less. Stress compounds the problem. It

is a vicious cycle: greater stress increases the clogging and constriction of the coronary arteries, and clogged and constricted
arteries are more reactive to stress. Even the muscles of the heart
can begin to constrict, causing damage to itself.

Fight or Flight

Experts talk about two ways that we respond to stress: the first
is called active coping, and it refers to the fight-or-flight response.
For example, you are driving in traffic and someone cuts you
off. You slam on the brakes and nearly miss becoming part of an
ugly accident. Your physical body's response is immediate and
complex. Put in simple terms, chemicals such as adrenaline and
changes in your sympathetic nervous system trigger several
events: an increase in breathing, blood pressure, and heart rate;
constriction of arteries; an increase in blood cholesterol and
other fats; and thickening of the blood. All these changes are
necessary preparations for possible injury, and they happen
automatically in your physical body.

At the same time, your inner emotional body may be express-
ing fear and heightened awareness, as well as many other possible emotions, during the crisis. When traffic clears and you are
out of danger, your physical body seems to return to normal fairly
quickly. But what about your inner emotional body? If you are
communicating with both your bodies, perhaps you would talk
to your inner body and console it; reassure it that you both are
still alive and well, that you appreciate how important it is to
take care of yourself, and acknowledge its fear and anxiety about
injury or death.

Vigilance

The second type of response to stress is called long-term monitoring, or vigilance. This refers to what happens when you are unable to let go of a stress reaction. This may be due to continual external pressures, such as an abusive spouse, a demanding boss, or caring for a seriously ill loved one; or it may be due to a constant internal reaction, such as continuing to mentally replay a near collision or a hostile confrontation. Your physical and emotional bodies continue in a state of low-grade chronic alarm as though the threat is still going on. Your emotional body feels fearful, angry, and in imminent danger even if the triggering event is well past. Your physical body does not go back to normal; instead, many of the most damaging changes brought about by the "fight or flight" response remain, such as high blood fats and increased blood pressure. Overweight can be a reaction to problems of every kind; the body adds fat for protection.

You can see how this second type of response creates unrelenting stress for both bodies, which then becomes a big risk factor for heart disease. The very conditions that contribute to arterial blockages and increase the likelihood of plaque formation — artery constriction, thickening of the blood, and greater amounts of cholesterol in the blood — are the same conditions that prevail under severe and constant stress. It is important to note, also, that it doesn't matter whether the stress is real, such as the near-miss accident described above, or imagined, such as constant worry about losing one's job; the same physical and emotional responses occur.

Type A and Your Heart

Decades ago, everyone was talking about the connection between heart disease and being a so-called Type A personality — one who is driven, competitive, and hostile, among other traits. Subsequent studies failed to find any connection between this personality type and risk of heart disease; however, when researchers looked at the individual characteristics, they found a definite relationship between heart disease and hostility, suppressed anger, and the need to be in control. The lack of control, especially, seems to trigger reactions in the nervous and hormonal systems that can lead to cardiovascular disease.

Social Support

Another important factor in how we respond to stress is our level of social support. People who have a high degree of social support have less risk of developing heart disease, even if other risk factors, such as smoking or obesity, are also present. Major life changes such as moving, changing jobs, divorce, and so on are often blamed for causing stress damage. However, it seems that those who have stronger ties to family and friends have more protection from the adverse effects of such life changes.

When you learn to manage stress more effectively with Yoga techniques, a balance develops between your physical and emotional bodies that helps lift yourself out of the self-absorption, depression, hostility, and fear that often accompany constant stress. To add to the problem, those who are under constant stress often medicate themselves with nicotine, alcohol and drugs; they don't eat well; they are more sedentary; and they don't rest well. Learning to manage stress helps your physical and emotional bodies to feel relaxed, empowered, and well; moreover, you feel stronger and better motivated to follow a healthy lifestyle.

How Yoga Helps

Yoga techniques have long been recognized as effective stress-coping tools. Regular daily practice of Yoga techniques helps your two bodies recover from stress events more quickly; you also learn to quiet your mind so that you can become aware of early warning signs of poor stress-coping — such as low frustration tolerance, excessive anxiety, shortness of breath, and so on. Practicing Yoga regularly, using the program outlined in this book, will help you recognize when you are unable to let go of stress and teach you ways to bring your physical and emotional bodies back into balance, giving your heart a big boost of protection. Stress reactions are usually caused by fear. Most people react to stress with only one-half of their being, the physical body. When you learn to pull in the support of both the physical and emotional/spiritual bodies in all your decisions, you gain full strength. Stress, then, cannot remain for long when faced by a balanced, united person using full capacity to deal with all problems and joys.

Chapter 3

How Yoga Can Improve Heart Health

The program for heart health presented in this book is designed to help you prevent or regress heart disease by learning to manage stress, reduce your cholesterol count, lose weight if necessary, improve blood flow in your coronary arteries, and build a healthy, strong heart. You will gain a greater sense of well-being, increase your strength for daily activities and overall disease resistance, and learn to see yourself not as a victim of disease but as a person who has the tools, courage, and confidence to get well and stay that way.

Our program teaches a lifestyle change: If you follow our guidelines, you will think differently, move differently, relax, breathe, and even eat differently. By making these techniques and ideas a part of your everyday life, you will have a much greater chance of maintaining your independence and reducing your risk for coronary artery disease.

This is a six-part program based on traditional Yoga techniques. Among the techniques presented to you in this book are physical exercises, breathing techniques, meditation training, fantasy exercises, attention to diet, awareness of ethics, and a special contemplation exercise to practice while doing moderate, briskly paced exercise. Here are some of the ways these techniques work:

• **EXERCISE.** The Yogic school of exercise, called asans, was developed for the body to maintain balanced mental and physical health. Yoga asans apply pressure to specific points, which affect different glands in the body. This helps the body to stay strong and totally balanced. This glandular pressure also promotes the release of the chemicals, called endorphins, that cause feelings of well-being in the brain. This aspect of Yoga practice can be very helpful in relieving depression, anxiety, and insomnia. Yoga asans help to improve strength, flexibility, vitality, posture, and muscle tone, which will help you feel and look better. The road to health lies in your own body. Regular Yoga practice builds your body's resistance to the negative effects of stress and allows you to recover more quickly from stressful events.

• **BREATHING.** Yoga breathing techniques nourish your inner body by helping to reduce anxiety and depression and create calm, clear, and creative thinking. The ancient Yoga teachers describe a mysterious way that breathing techniques cleanse the nervous system, making its full function available for body needs. Breathing exercises also develop a depth of sensitivity which is very helpful in dealing with your inner emotional spiritual body. The effects are especially noticeable when you spend some extra time trying to begin a new relationship with your inner self.

Many people first come to Yoga in order to reduce their stress responses. Even a little daily practice of Yoga breathing techniques can help you learn how to cope with the inevitable anxieties of life, especially if you are undergoing the additional stresses of coping with the fear of heart disease or trying to lose weight. Many people report that concentrating on their breath helps reduce anxiety as it relaxes the body.

• **MEDITATION.** Yoga meditation techniques increase self-awareness and augment the balanced, calming effects of exercises and breathing techniques. In the practice of meditation, the physical body is quieted and all inner conversation is silenced for a short time. This allows the intuitive voice, which is the language of the inner emotional body, to speak. This intuitive voice is the gateway for expression that the inner spiritual body seeks, and it provides comfort from within. Meditation is one way to acknowledge your inner emotional body. Meditation also gives both your bodies a daily complete rest. In this quiet state, your entire physical body relaxes, similar to deep sleep, and it can have a wonderful healing effect on the body's inner emotional strength.

• **FANTASY.** Guided Yoga Fantasy techniques help you envision a healthy heart from within. Fantasy also enhances self-esteem. Through practice of these techniques, which you can use throughout the day during many activities of daily life, you will learn that your inner thoughts and feelings determine your image of yourself and how you face and behave in the world. Regular practice of these Fantasy exercises will help you build and sustain a new image of yourself as you wish to be.

• **MODERATE EXERCISE.** Moderate-intensity exercise helps to improve cardiovascular fitness, burn calories, and build muscle. In our program, we teach you how to perform this moderate exercise at your own pace and with a Yogic mind of centered attention: a quiet meditative focus on your inner self. The best all-around moderate-intensity exercise is walking; it can be done by almost anyone, and it can be done safely while centering your attention on one of the contemplation exercises introduced in Chapter 8. Walking can be done outside in any safe environment, or inside on any suitable treadmill. Other forms of exercise that will work with this technique are swimming and riding a stationary bicycle.

• DIET. A diet for a healthy heart is essentially a well-balanced diet emphasizing whole foods and fresh fruits and vegetables, and reducing cholesterol and fats. Depending on your current cholesterol level and your doctor's recommendations, we help you choose how to regulate the components of your diet to achieve optimal results. Many people with heart problems need to lose weight; this chapter also provides some tips for losing weight at a slow but steady rate. An important section offers recommendations for changing your taste preferences in foods to emphasize healthier choices while not giving up enjoyment.

These are the basic components of our Yoga program for heart health. Before starting to teach you the routine itself, I'd like to discuss the role of ethics in Yoga practice, and introduce you to a wonderful motivational technique that has worked well for many of my students.

Ethics in Yoga

Many times, Yoga is misunderstood as religious. Yoga is not a religion; it is a way to find yourself, a joining, a bridge to the unknown parts of yourself. The science of Yoga provides tools that can be used by people of any faith or background to enhance their lives. Throughout this book, I've used the term "emotional/spiritual" to refer to your inner body; I do not use the word "spiritual" in a religious sense but rather as a way to indicate that something else within you, besides your familiar physical and mental processes, is also deeply involved in your health and well-being. This inner self is often unknown to us until we learn how to pay attention to it, and Yoga techniques are a way to welcome the participation of this inner being.

One of the most important aspects of Yoga is the practice of ethics. Yoga philosophy teaches that ethics are the safe gateway to the inner self. In other words, you can fully experience the participation of your emotional/spiritual body only with the help of an awareness and practice of ethical behavior. Yoga holds great reverence for life, and for this reason, the ethic of Nonviolence becomes its mainstay. In the view of Yoga, the ethic of Nonviolence applies first and foremost to yourself. This is especially important when dealing with disease. Whether you have already been diagnosed with heart problems, or you simply want to reduce your risk, making the lifestyle changes presented in this book are a way of beginning this important practice of Nonviolence.

I believe that if you learn to connect to your inner emotional/spiritual body through the practice of ethics, particularly Nonviolence, you will grow to enjoy the lifestyle changes that health demands. The longer you practice, the more you will become able to see your dietary changes and other techniques not as harsh disciplines but as helpful, enjoyable practices that will free you from disease and dependence. In one of the most well-known Yogic texts, the *Bhagavad Gita*, there is a phrase that explains this phenomenon perfectly. It says, in talking about establishing regular practice, that it seems "like poison in the beginning, but like nectar in the end." When you first begin your heart health program, it may seem like a lot of effort and may even be a little uncomfortable, especially if you are unused to exercise or have followed a traditional American diet for many years. With practice, however, you will find that your Yoga routine becomes habitual and quite enjoyable as you gain strength and health. Great joy comes from emotional balance.

Many experts in the field of psychology have discussed the fact that humans have an innate tendency toward self-annihilation ("thanatos") that constantly battles with the body's natural instinct for survival ("eros"). You can see this in people who turn to drugs, alcohol, and other self-violent behaviors in an attempt to escape from pain, disease, or depression, not realizing that they are not only making their condition worse, but in reality hastening their own death.

Yoga philosophy recognizes these opposing forces and teaches students to be aware of both tendencies as they make choices in life. The study of ethics in Yoga is the best way to recognize when you are being violent toward yourself and offer you the ability to choose to behave differently. The *Gita* says, "You are your own best friend and your own worst enemy." By consciously choosing a healthy lifestyle while acknowledging the other choices that you have left behind, you will develop increasing strength that will carry you through anything that you do in life. Depression usually hides the fact that you have a choice in what you do.

Regular daily practice of the Yoga program outlined in this book will prepare your physical body to join with your inner emotional body without pain or upset. The results show very quickly. You should feel the difference in just two or three days. It is hard to describe this change, because the body does not change quickly, but the feelings that accompany regular practice are so pleasant that you won't want to give it up; these feelings reflect the participation of your inner body in the healing process. The two bodies at the board meeting can finally talk to each other as the rift of separateness heals, giving you the full power to be what you want to be.

Those who take up the practice of Yoga in this nonviolent way rarely ever stop. Thousands of people who have always hated to exercise and have been unable to maintain a happy daily discipline now look forward to their daily practice of Yoga because it allows the inner emotional body to join the physical in exertion. You will never fear it; in fact, you will really miss your practices if you don't do them. You don't have to go to a class to achieve this effect; practicing at home alone with this book, or with a class videotape such as our "Basic Yoga" (see Resources), will give you wonderful results.

A regular daily routine of Yoga exercises, breathing, meditation, and fantasy, even if it lasts only a few minutes, will produce happy, comforting expression from the inner emotional body. When this happens, healing begins.

The Wrist Tape Technique

Now I am going to introduce you to a wonderful motivational tool that you can use to help you succeed in your program for heart health. My students have great luck with this technique, which they use when they want to change something in their behavior. It is extremely successful in the practice of ethics or any other behavioral change that you wish to attempt.

Let's say you want to become more aware of how often during the day you do or say something that is hurtful to yourself — in other words, something contrary to the lifestyle changes you are trying to make in order to reduce your risk of heart disease. To try the wrist tape exercise, simply place a small piece of nonirritating tape, such as first aid-type adhesive tape, a Band-Aid, or painter's masking tape, on the inside of your wrist or on a watch band. Every time you notice yourself doing or saying something that is violent to yourself, make a mark on the tape. For instance, if you look in the mirror and say "I look awful," that would be a violent thought; if you are trying to cut cholesterol in your diet but you eat a fatty dessert anyway, that would be a violent act. At the end of the day, paste the tape on your refrigerator door. By the week's end you will see a row of tapes indicating how you have progressed in acting on your new vision of yourself. The tapes will show you that violence to yourself is showing a pattern.

Using a Wrist Tape to Practice Nonviolence

Here is what one student wrote to me about her practice of this technique: "When I caught myself in a violent thought and made a mark, it was as if I was able to let it go, instead of grinding and grinding about whatever it was that was upsetting me. I know this connection is nebulous, but somehow it helped me to see that nothing is outside of myself; that all those things that I thought were out there upsetting me were actually reflections of my own self — my unconscious self that I tend to forget to talk to, even though I've been trying every day to take time out to give it voice. It's made me take another look at the way I've been trying to run my life."

This practice promotes great respect for yourself because it reflects the great effort you are putting into your lifestyle change. When you are able to perceive the effort clearly, you will be able to really congratulate your inner emotional spiritual body for its support in the process. This will begin to bring you together with your emotional self in a nonviolent process that will develop a friendly support within yourself for what you want to do.

Be Kind to Yourself

Now you are ready to begin our complete Yoga Program for Heart Health. Don't worry if you cannot do the complete routine all at once. In fact, if you have not exercised in a long time, it will be much more beneficial to start slowly, doing only three exercises each day and adding techniques as you gain strength and stamina. Always try to practice a little every day. This daily consistency will give momentum to your efforts and result in quicker and longer lasting results.

Here is a suggested schedule for the first week, incorporating each of the six parts of our program, illustrating how to increase your practice gradually over several weeks:

Exercise

> *All warm-ups, plus three exercises (add 1-2 new exercises each week as you gain strength and interest).*

Breathing

> *3 Complete Breaths (add 3 repetitions each week until you reach one minute total; next try the Cooling Breath*

technique and build up to one minute over several weeks; then add the Alternate Nostril Breath and the Soft Bellows Breath in the same way. Your total practice of breathing techniques at one sitting will never exceed four minutes. Of course, you can practice breathing techniques at other times of the day as described in Chapter 5. It is a wonderful way to pass time waiting for appointments or delays).

Meditation

5 minutes (add 3 minutes per week until you reach 20 minutes — about six weeks; stay at this length of time indefinitely, or continue to 30 minutes in 3-minute intervals as before).

Fantasy

"Creating a Vision of a Healthy Heart." (Practice this every day for one week, then try a new Fantasy exercise the same way during the following week and the week after. Then alternate techniques as you wish, or practice them combined with your activity program as described in Chapter 8).

Walking Contemplation

5-10 minutes per day. (Add 5 minutes per week until you reach 30 minutes per day).

Diet

In the first week, choose just one change to make in your diet; for example, switch from 2% milk to fat-free; or, instead of meat for a main course one day, try a dish made from a soy protein substitute. See Chapter 10 for more suggestions. Continue making a small change each week until you are following the entire recommended dietary plan happily.

Some of my students enjoy recording their progress in a chart form. If you like, create a chart or a journal that records your goals for each of the six parts of the program for each week, and include a space to write in how you met your goals, what you experienced during your Fantasy exercises or while meditating, and how you felt about yourself every day. Here is a sample:

Week 1
Exercise

Goal — *warm-ups and 3 exercises.*

Result — *warm-ups only for 2 days, then added the Standing Sun Pose. Felt a little stiffness in the back of my legs, but it went away by the end of the week.*

Breathing

Goal — *3 Complete Breath exercises*

Result — *Loved this technique! Found myself doing it while waiting in the doctor's office Wednesday. Helped me feel less nervous.*

Meditation

Goal — *5 minutes*

Result — *Felt like I was just lying there thinking about my "to do" list. About the third day, felt myself stop talking to myself for a few seconds. By the end of the week, I almost fell asleep.*

Fantasy

Goal — *"Vision of a Healthy Heart"*

Result — *Had trouble seeing anything but a vision of myself helpless and sick at first. About halfway through the week, had an experience where I felt my heart full of light and strength.*

Walking

Goal — *5-10 minutes*

Result — *Got overenthusiastic the first day: walked around the neighborhood for about a half hour — felt sore the next day. Walked 5 minutes anyway. Felt better. Missed only one day this week.*

Diet

Goal — *make one small change in diet*

Result — *Decided to try milk in my coffee instead of cream. Succeeded every day except Sunday.*

Always maintain a constant, friendly approach with yourself, reminding yourself that this is a lifetime change that slowly and steadily will build solid supporting blocks of health, strength, and happiness with yourself and your new way of living.

Chapter 4

Yoga Exercise for Heart Health

In this chapter you will find a complete Yoga exercise routine especially designed to be helpful for heart health. The routine is organized so that the easiest exercises are presented first, so start at the beginning. If you have not exercised in a long time, I suggest that you begin by practicing only the warm-ups (pages 57-70) and then three additional exercises. Add two or three exercises each week until you are able to practice the full routine.

How to Practice Yoga Exercises for Best Results

Breathing

It may be tempting to plunge right in and just follow the pictures, but if you do you will miss the important instructions about how to breathe during the exercise. Breathing is a crucial element of Yoga exercise, and each pose or movement has a particular breathing pattern that contributes greatly to its effect. Read once completely through the instructions before beginning, in order to be sure you are breathing correctly as well as to avoid injury.

Always breathe through your nose, both inhaling and exhaling. If you concentrate on the steamlike sound of your breath as you move through the routine, you will notice a wonderful silence in your mind that will naturally lead you into a very restful meditation. (See Chapter 5, p. 124, for how to make the steamlike sound with your breath and how to breathe more freely if one side of your nose is blocked.)

The exercises have been laid out in a sequence from standing to seated to lying down. The transition between exercises is often where concentration is lost. Try to keep your attention on your breath throughout the entire routine, moving smoothly from one exercise to another with graceful movement.

Most exercises are a series of movements matched with either an inhalation or an exhalation and a brief hold at the top and bottom of the breath, all done to a count of three. This focuses and settles your mind on the proper position of body, breath, and mind. Don't count so slowly that you find yourself gasping for breath. There is no specific speed for this three-count, such as three seconds; the counting is simply to focus your attention. Count faster if you need to, to avoid getting winded. As you get more proficient, slow down the count.

Work at Your Own Pace

Yoga exercises should not hurt. Be kind to your body! Move slowly and carefully, paying attention to how your body feels at all times. I can't stress enough how important it is to work at your own pace. As I mentioned previously, if you haven't exercised in a long time, don't try to do the entire routine all at once. In fact, it's probably a good idea to do only one repetition of each exercise the first few times you try it, just to make sure there is no movement that will aggravate a back condition or other physical problem you may not be aware of. When you feel confident, move on to three repetitions of each exercise.

As I've said previously in this book, the important thing is to practice at least three exercises every day. When you practice every day, your strength and endurance will gradually increase until you can do the entire routine. When you find that the exercises are becoming too easy, you can add more repetitions to give yourself more of a challenge.

Alternatively, if some of the exercises are too difficult, practice them at only half capacity until you become more proficient. Remember, Yoga is a nonviolent practice. If you haven't exercised in a while, you may experience some tightness in your joints and muscles, especially in the back of your legs when you practice forward-bending exercises. With daily practice, you will notice a big difference in your stretching ability in just a few weeks.

Most exercises call for about three to five repetitions. Always go at your own pace, remembering that Yoga works best in small steady increments.

Warm-ups

The first several exercises in your routine gradually introduce your body to the idea of exercising. They are simple stretches that work on the major muscle groups of the body, gently stretching the long muscles of the legs and back, gently bending the spine, increasing circulation, and loosening the joints of the shoulders, hips, and spine. Remember to breathe through your nose at all times and concentrate on the sound of the breath. Pay attention to how your body feels, and never do anything that causes pain. In the following routine, the warm-ups begin with the Shoulder Roll and end with the Easy Balance.

Stress is a pervasive force in our daily lives that can cause the physical body to fear movement because it is afraid of attack, no matter what the source, or whether it's justified or not. It's as if the body feels such a need for protection — especially if it has not exercised in a long time — that it carefully guards its movements so as not to be hurt. The Shoulder Roll and other warm-ups will help your body to gradually feel more relaxed about the movements that lie ahead in the routine so that it doesn't feel so frightened.

The B-complex vitamins and vitamin C are very important for helping support your body to manage stress responses, and calcium/magnesium helps muscles and nerves relax. See Chapter 9 for more information about how to be sure your diet includes enough of these nutrients.

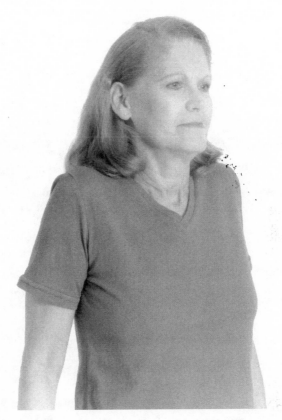

(1) Shoulder Roll

SHOULDER ROLL

Benefits: Loosens shoulder joints and upper back.

Breathe normally throughout this exercise. Stand with feet parallel and arms hanging loosely at your sides. Lift both shoulders up toward your ears (without bending your elbows) and rotate your shoulders in circles, first forward, then backward, at least five times in each direction (1). Keep your arms and hands hanging loosely.

Learning to relax at will is a vital skill for a Yoga student. Every exercise provides an opportunity to learn a different way to relax your body and mind. Sometimes the best relaxation comes after an exertion. In the Arm Circles, your heart and the rest of your respiratory and circulatory systems are energized, so your entire upper body feels flushed with life-giving blood that is packed with oxygen. Enhance the relaxed feeling by shaking out your arms and shoulders after this exercise.

Sometimes people who have trouble relaxing during the day also have trouble going to sleep at night or staying asleep. If this applies to you, try cutting out caffeinated beverages after 5 p.m. Practice a few warm-ups just before bed, and practice two or three Complete Breaths when you lie down. Try to think of nothing except the sound of your breath. Then meditate yourself to sleep with the "I Love You" technique (see page 143).

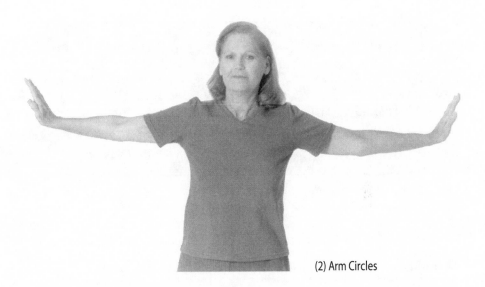

(2) Arm Circles

ARM CIRCLES

Benefits: Increases circulation; strengthens back and shoulders; improves range of motion of shoulders; limbers upper back, chest, and midback.

Stand with feet parallel. Lift your arms straight out to the sides, fingers flexed and palms facing outward (2). Maintaining this position, rotate your arms first in large, slow circles and then in small, faster circles, five to eight times in each direction. Breathe normally throughout. Finish by shaking out arms and shoulders.

> In this exercise, you are concentrating on the movement of just one part of your body. This is a wonderful opportunity to practice the quiet feeling that you are striving for in meditation. Stop all inner conversation with yourself, which will dilute the effect of the exercise. Instead, imagine, as you turn your head slowly, that your head is filled with a great silence.

NECK STRETCHES

Benefits: Releases tension in upper back and neck.

Cautions: If you have known disk problems or chronic pain or stiffness in your neck, check with your doctor before trying this exercise.

Start by gently bending your neck to the right and slightly forward, so your chin reaches down toward your collarbone. Place your left palm on your neck to monitor the stretch (3). Hold for several seconds, breathing normally. Repeat on the opposite side. Release, and gently turn your head from side to side.

If you have no neck problems, you may add a **Head Rotation**: Place your hands on your hips or let them hang straight down, and keep your shoulders relaxed. Gently bend your head to the left, bending your ear over your shoulder and being careful not to lift your shoulder up (4). Roll your head forward, chin toward your chest, and continue rolling your head over toward the right shoulder, then back slightly, then over to the left to complete the circle. Repeat, slowly, twice more to the left and then three times to the right. Keep shoulders relaxed at all times; the only parts of your body that should move are your head and neck.

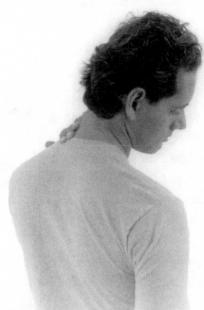

(3) Neck Stretches

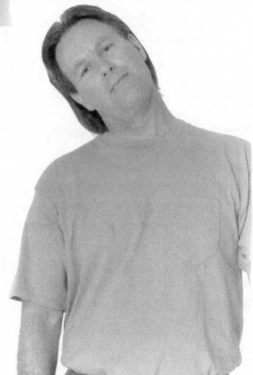

(4) Neck Stretches

The previous warm-ups focused on your upper body. With the Elbow Twist exercise, you will begin to feel the effects of improved circulation in your lower back, hips, and legs. Continue the mental exercise described for the Neck Stretches. Imagine yourself filled with a vast silence. Imagine the silence spreading throughout your entire body. You will feel a restful feeling of relief while you slowly twist from side to side. Your physical body will loosen up and begin to deepen the relaxation of back and shoulder muscles. Your emotional body will feel centered and focused.

ELBOW TWIST

Benefits: Limbers spine; improves respiration and posture.

Stand with feet a few inches apart, and be sure your back is straight. Raise your arms to chest height and place one hand on top of the other. Breathe in completely to a count of three while looking forward, hold for a count of three, then breathe out to a count of three as you slowly twist toward the left, leading with your left elbow. Look around to the left so your entire upper body is gently twisted (5), and hold for a count of three. Breathe in to a count of three as you return to the front. Breathe out and slowly twist to the right. Hold, then breathe in and return to the front. Repeat 2 to 5 times to each side, alternating.

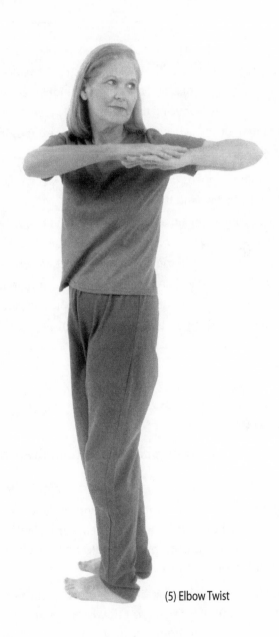

(5) Elbow Twist

My teacher Rama used to say that this simple exercise is the key to total body health. It uses all the major muscle groups, and affects the nervous, circulatory, glandular, and respiratory systems. Practicing this exercise will prevent the development of a swayback or hunchback. This exercise invites a mystical connection with the sun.

Nothing happens in the physical world without first happening in the mind. If you want to build a chair, for example, you first have to fantasize the chair in your mind; then you pick up the saw and hammer to build the chair. Similarly, when you practice Yoga exercises, you attain best results if you fantasize the changes you want to see in your body. As you practice the Full Bend, visualize your body stretching out until it becomes taut and lean and brave.

FULL BEND AND HOLD
(Paschimottanasan Prep.)

Benefits: Releases tension in upper back and neck; helps to reduce a large stomach.

Cautions: If you start to feel faint while bending forward, bend only halfway down, but still be sure to let your head, arms, and hands hang forward loosely when you breathe out. Hold on to a chair back or railing with one hand to protect from falling.

Stand with feet parallel, a few inches apart. Breathe out completely. Breathe in to a count of three as you slowly raise your arms up and out to your sides, parallel to the floor (6). Stretch back a little as you hold your breath in for a count of three, then breathe out to a count of three as you slowly bend forward, leading with your hands, until you are as far for-

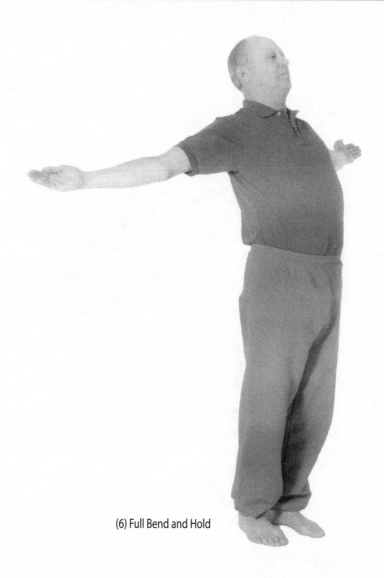

(6) Full Bend and Hold

ward as possible. Let your whole body go limp and hold your breath out
(7). Now breathe in and slowly come back up, bringing your arms out to
the sides again. Continue to breathe in as you straighten up and breathe
out as you bend forward, matching your breath to your movement and
using the three-count as previously instructed. Repeat 3 to 5 times.

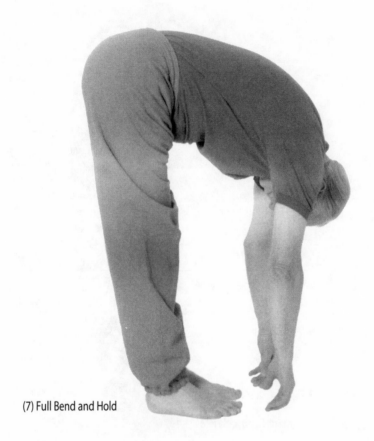

(7) Full Bend and Hold

After the last repetition, breathe out and come forward once again, but let your arms relax toward the floor and hold the position, breathing naturally. If you can reach the floor comfortably, let your fingers curl slightly. Just go limp and relax. Let your head hang so your neck stretches. Don't hold your breath. Hold for several seconds, then slowly stand up.

You will like this movement. It is an easy exercise to begin with if your body is afraid to move because of pain. It helps give strength to your hands and arms, and you will enjoy the ability to balance on your toes for a moment or two, which is all that is needed. If you are afraid to go up on your toes for fear of falling, hold on to a sturdy chair or kitchen countertop first with one hand, then the other, in order to exercise each side equally.

EASY BALANCE

Benefits: Improves respiration; oxygenates blood; strengthens ankles and calves; improves balance.

Standing with feet parallel and arms at sides, breathe out. Staring at one spot to help maintain balance, breathe in completely to a count of three as you stretch up on your toes and press your fists into your midriff (8). Be sure you are not pressing into your rib cage, but directly below it. Hold for a count of three, then breathe out to a count of three as you relax, lowering your arms and heels. Rest. Repeat 3 times.

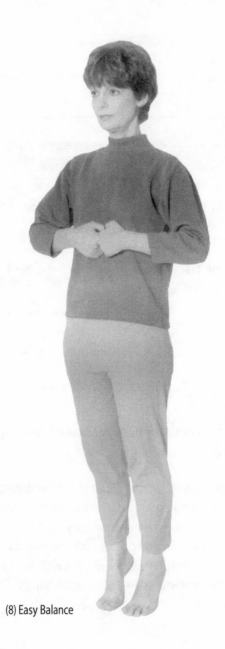

(8) Easy Balance

Dance rituals are practiced by indigenous peoples throughout the world to celebrate the cycles of life and the seasons. We all enjoy the grace of a dancer, and this pose will help you develop the graceful movement that is displayed by dancers of all cultures. Picture yourself as a dancer. Be poised and confident as you balance. This exercise is very helpful to do before a stressful meeting. It will give you quiet confidence.

DANCER POSE (Natarajasan)

Benefits: Strengthens lower back and lumbar vertebrae; stretches and strengthens hips and thighs; improves balance, poise, and concentration; removes phlegm and opens the nasal passages; improves memory; relieves sluggishness and depression.

From a standing position, bend your left leg and grasp your foot with the opposite hand (9). Throughout the exercise, steady yourself by fixing your gaze on one spot on the wall in front of you. Slowly move into the completed Dancer Pose by raising your free arm straight up toward the ceiling next to your ear and pulling your lifted leg up and back as far as possible without strain (10). Keep your supporting leg straight and keep your gaze focused on one spot. Breathe in to a count of three and hold your breath in for a count of three.

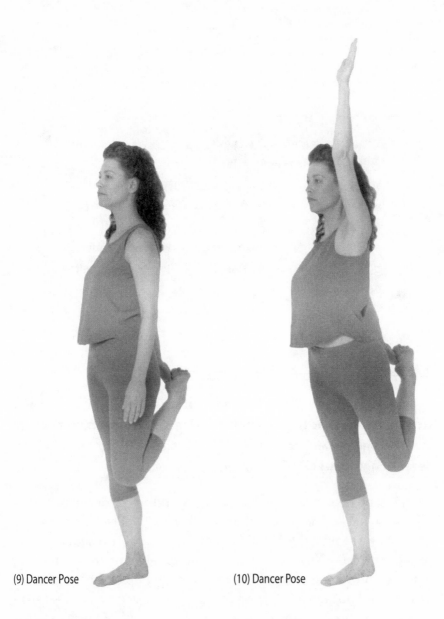

(9) Dancer Pose   (10) Dancer Pose

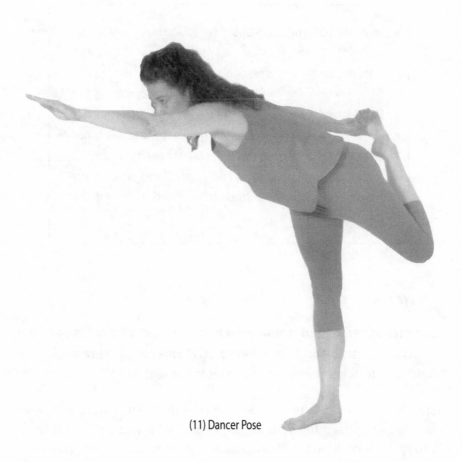

(11) Dancer Pose

Maintaining your gaze, slowly breathe out to a count of three as you lower your body into the extended position (11). Keep your lifted leg as far up and back as possible. Your free arm extends straight ahead. Your supporting leg remains straight. Stare at one spot for balance. Don't strain. Hold for a count of three, then breathe in to a count of three as you come back to a standing position. Switch sides. This exercise is done only once on each side.

I believe that emotional upset can lodge in the body, particularly the large muscles such as those in the thighs and arms, increasing stress responses and muscle tension even if you are not consciously aware of it. Exercises such as the Thigh Stretch can help you to gradually let go of emotional tension as these long muscles are gently stretched. Another place in the body that holds emotional stress is the respiratory muscles. Breathe deeply and slowly as you perform this exercise to increase the stress relief and thus reduce the stress on your heart.

THIGH STRETCH

Benefits: Stretches and strengthens hamstrings, groin muscles, and hip joints; increases blood circulation to pelvis; may improve reproductive function; stretches nerves and muscles in the legs.

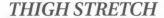

Start by kneeling on the floor. Stretch your right leg forward with your foot flat, and straighten your left leg in back with toes tucked under. (If you find this position too strenuous, you may rest the knee of your back leg on the floor.) Breathe out completely, then breathe in to a count of three as you stretch forward, arching your back and looking up to increase the stretch on both legs (12). Hold for a count of three. Breathe out to a count of three as you sit back, straightening both legs and bending your head forward toward your right knee (13). Hold for a count of three. Repeat three times each side.

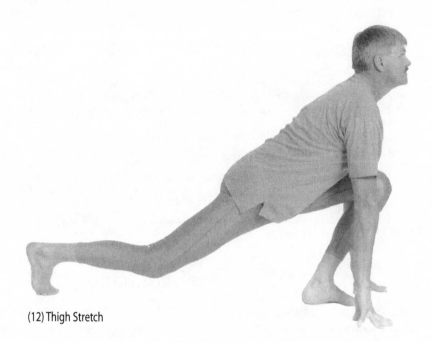

(12) Thigh Stretch

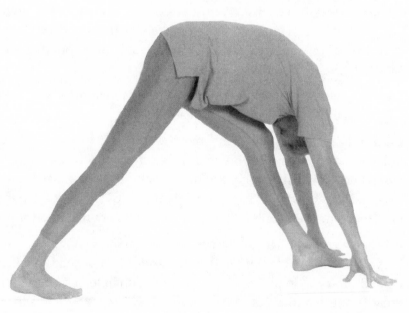

(13) Thigh Stretch

> There is a reason this exercise is called the "Sun Pose": it brings radiant, all-around health, just as the sun is the earth's source for nourishment and growth. The best way to practice this exercise is to visualize the sun as you raise your arms and breathe in deeply. Hold this image in your mind's eye as you complete the exercise, then rest. The radiant, life-giving properties of the sun will fill your heart and body.

STANDING SUN POSE (Padahasthasan)

Benefits: Improves functioning of digestive and circulatory systems; exercises heart and lungs; limbers and strengthens legs and back.

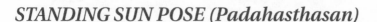

Stand with feet parallel. Keep your knees straight but not locked. Breathe out. Breathe in to a count of three as you raise your arms in a wide circle to the sides (14) and overhead. Stretch and look up at your hands (15). Hold your breath in for a count of three.

Breathe out to a count of three as you bend forward from the waist, keeping your hands together and your head between your arms (16).

Grasp your ankles or calves firmly, bend your elbows, tuck your chin, and pull your torso toward your legs (17). Be sure to pull by bending your elbows instead of straining your lower back. Keep your knees straight and hold your breath out for a count of three. [NOTE: If you have back or neck problems, bend only halfway down, and do not pull your torso in.]

Release and breathe in to a count of three as you slowly straighten, bringing your arms in a wide circle to the sides and over your head again. Look up and stretch as in photo 15. Hold your breath in for a count of three. Breathe out to a count of three as you slowly lower your arms to your sides. Repeat three times.

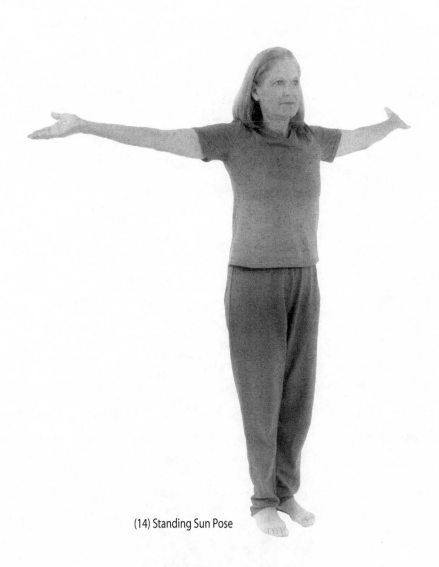

(14) Standing Sun Pose

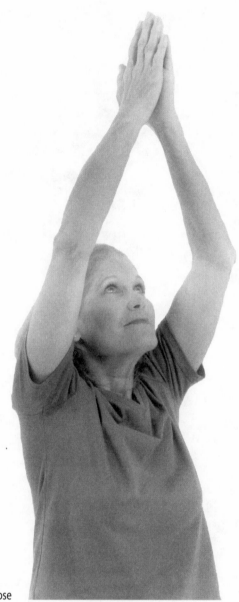

(15) Standing Sun Pose

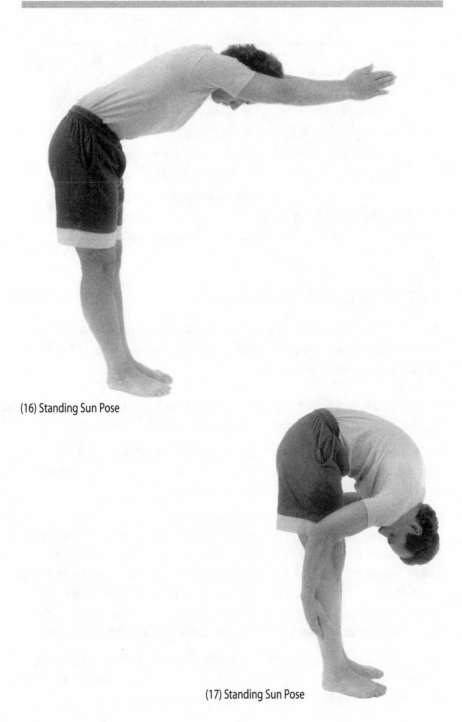

(16) Standing Sun Pose

(17) Standing Sun Pose

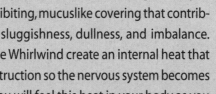

In Yoga, the nervous system is often pictured figuratively as covered with an inhibiting, mucuslike covering that contributes to feelings of sluggishness, dullness, and imbalance. Exercises such as the Whirlwind create an internal heat that clears away this obstruction so the nervous system becomes bright and active. You will feel this heat in your body as you practice, and probably notice a more positive and energetic state of mind.

THE WHIRLWIND (Nauli)

Benefits: Compresses internal abdominal organs; strengthens abdominal muscles; reduces body fat. Many people feel a very pleasant warmth building up during the exercise.

Caution: Do not practice the standing variation if you have a lower back problem, as it puts greater strain on your back when standing.

Because this exercise requires you to hold your breath out for quite a while, it can be a bit strenuous until you learn it. Be sure to read through the entire set of instructions before beginning.

Note: If your abdominal muscles are weak, try the **Easy Sit-up** for a few weeks before attempting the Whirlwind: Lying on your back with knees bent and feet flat, place your hands on your legs and breathe out. Breathe in as you curl up, sliding your hands toward your knees. Breathe out and lower. Practice this exercise for a few weeks until your strength increases. When you can easily do 15-20 sit-ups in a row, you should be able to perform the Rising Breath and Whirlwind exercises without straining.

Begin with a technique called the **Rising Breath** (Uddhyana). It is very beneficial to health, strength, and brightness of mind, and it will help you master the movement needed for the Whirlwind.

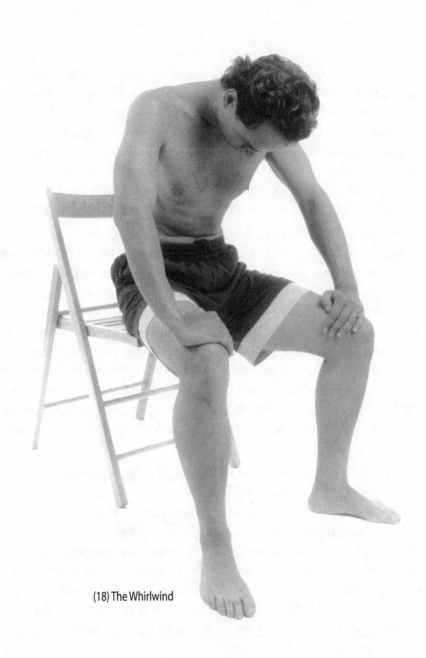

(18) The Whirlwind

Sitting on the very edge of a sturdy chair, separate your knees and "plant" your feet flat on the floor. Place your hands just above your knees, pointing in. Tuck your chin into your throat. Begin by taking five deep and strong Belly Breaths (see Chapter 5, p. 125), then breathe out forcefully and completely. Be sure all the air is expelled. Holding your breath out, suck in your abdominal muscles back toward your spine and up toward your diaphragm (18). Hold for just a moment, then release your stomach muscles, release your breath, breathe in, and relax. Relax and rest until your breath returns to normal. Practice three repetitions.

When you feel relatively proficient in this movement, go on to the Whirlwind *(Nauli)*, which is a similar contraction that you learn to move from side to side in your abdominal cavity: Begin in the same seated position, with chin tucked into your chest. Breathe in deeply, then breathe out forcefully and completely. Hold your breath out and suck in your abdominal muscles back toward your spine and up toward your diaphragm. Press down slightly on your left leg and you will feel the left side of your abdominal wall contract. Now press equally with both hands and then with the right hand only. You will feel the abdominal contraction move across the front of your belly from left to right. Now equalize the pressure on your knees and slowly let your belly relax. Relax your breath and your entire body.

For daily practice, start with one repetition and work up to five. Each repetition consists of left to center to right and back to center. Don't hold any of the positions for more than a few seconds. Always relax completely between repetitions. As you get stronger, you can do up to three cycles during each repetition. Be gentle with yourself. Rest immediately if you feel dizziness or discomfort. Note: for a more challenging variation of this exercise, practice in a standing, half-squat position, with hands on separated knees (19). In this position, the pose has very powerful effects on the reproductive system as the abdominal muscles are pulled in and up.

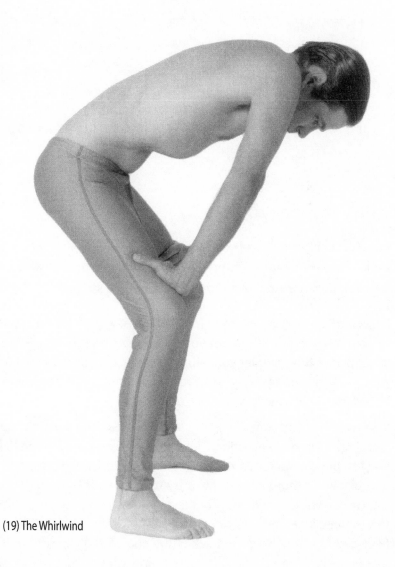

(19) The Whirlwind

This exercise looks like a rest pose, but it is actually a very powerful technique for bringing all the parts of yourself into harmony. Gather yourself together internally as you strongly compress your body as much as you can without discomfort. Stop inner conversation. Try to stay silent in your mind.

BABY POSE (Virasan Var.)

Benefits: Limbers and relaxes lower back; improves circulation to the brain and pelvic region; improves reproductive and digestive system functioning; improves respiration; reduces large stomach.

Kneel and sit on your feet. Bend forward, keeping your hips on your feet, so your forehead or the top of your head rests on the floor. Bring your arms to your sides and let your elbows fall outward slightly so that your shoulders relax completely (20). Breathe naturally and relax your entire body. Hold for as long as you can comfortably.

If you cannot bend completely forward while keeping your hips on your feet due to a large midsection, high blood pressure, or extreme discomfort, just bend as far forward as you can or rest your head on folded arms or a pillow. It's more important to try to keep your hips on your heels than to rest your head on the floor. If your knees or hips are too stiff to do this exercise kneeling, you can sit in a straight chair with feet flat on the floor and hips touching the back of the chair. Simply bend forward so that your head hangs over your knees and your arms hang loosely at your sides (21). Be sure to relax the back of your neck.

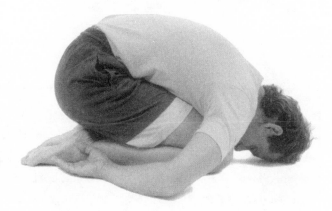

(20) Baby Pose

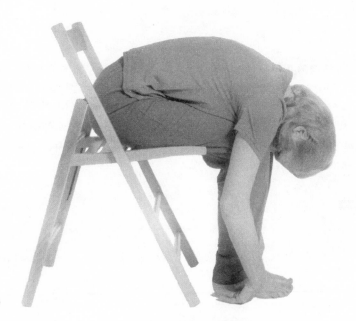

(21) Baby Pose

Do you remember the fairy tale about the Frog Prince? Yogis believe that myths and fairy tales are based on the universal experiences of archetypal transformation that occur when people begin to change their outlook about who and what they are. As you practice this simple Yoga exercise, visualize the lowly frog turning into a luminous prince or princess and visualize yourself blooming into a new vision of health and strength.

FROG POSE

Sit straight, either in a chair or on the floor on your heels. Place your hands on your knees. Breathe in to a count of three as you arch your back and look up, leaning forward slightly (22). Hold for a count of three. Breathe out to a count of three as you bend the opposite way, rounding your back and tucking your chin into your chest (23). Hold for a count of three. Repeat twice more.

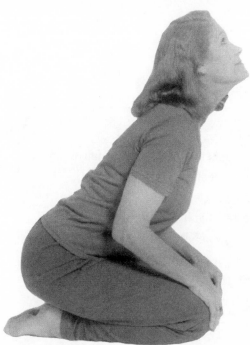

(22) Frog Pose

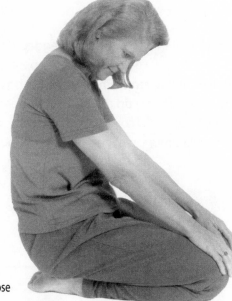

(23) Frog Pose

The muscles on the sides of the torso and rib cage are not often used, yet they are essential to correct and full respiration. This exercise will stretch and relax these muscles, improving the health and efficiency of your lungs and heart. As you practice exercises that use muscles that are not familiar, try to move your awareness in new directions as well. Try to imagine the muscles you are using as you practice this exercise, fantasizing them lengthening, filling with fresh blood and oxygen, and becoming stronger.

SIDE STRETCH

Sit straight in a chair or cross-legged on the floor. Let your arms relax at your sides. Take a deep breath in to a count of three as you bend toward your right side, stretching your right arm down toward the floor and bending your left arm up and over your head (24). Hold for a count of three. Breathe out to a count of three as you return to your starting position. Repeat 3 times on each side, alternating.

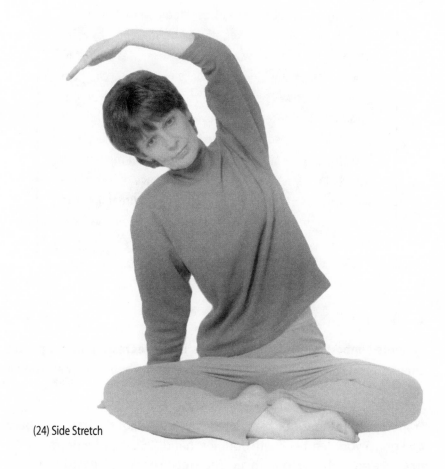

(24) Side Stretch

According to my teachers, Yoga exercise and meditation allow the body to set its own correct heart rate. Each person has a unique pattern of heart conditioning that he or she can bring to maximum strength and health simply by practicing Yoga asans. As few as three Yoga exercises every day, practiced correctly, along with daily meditation, can help bring all the body's systems into balance. The health of your cardiovascular system is improved in other ways through Yoga practice: specifically, in exercises such as the Camel Pose, the precise stretching and compression movements work to increase the flexibility and resilience of blood vessels as well as muscle and connective tissue. Breathing and meditation techniques help to relax the fine muscles that can constrict blood vessels.

CAMEL POSE (Ustrasan)

Benefits: Limbers entire spine and pelvis; improves respiration; improves circulation in spinal column; stretches and strengthens upper and lower thigh and knees.

From a kneeling position, separate your knees slightly, arch your back and grasp your left heel with your left hand (25). Breathe normally. Do this once on each side to warm up. Then reach back and grasp both heels (26). Push your hips forward as far as possible without straining. Let your head gently fall back as you breathe out to a count of three (unless you have known disk problems or chronic upper back or neck pain or stiffness, in which case keep your head up). Hold for a count of three, then breathe in to a count of three as you release. Rest.

Variation: If you are unable to grasp both heels at once, do the exercise once on each side in position 25 instead.

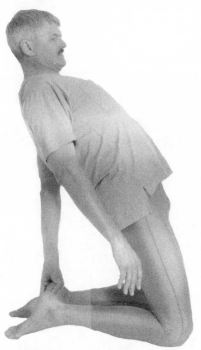

(25) Camel Pose

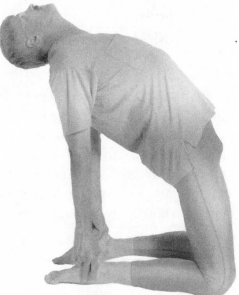

(26) Camel Pose

Balance poses are wonderful indicators of the general health and strength of your nervous system. This exercise may take extra strength to learn. Work up to it slowly, and you will find that your eventual success will help lift any depression that you may feel, and will fill you with confidence. The B complex vitamins are also important for a healthy nervous system. Read Chapter 9 for more about how to be sure your diet is complete.

CROW POSE (Kakasan)

Benefits: Strengthens hands, wrists, arms, and shoulders; improves balance and circulation.

Cautions: Always have a support near you, such as a chair, to avoid falling.

Squat on your toes, separate your knees, and place your hands on the floor between your knees about a foot apart. Bend your elbows and place the inside joint of your knees on your elbows (you'll have to lift your hips slightly to do this). Carefully lean forward, resting your bent knees on the back of your elbows, until your feet come off the floor (27). Breathe out and stare at one spot on the floor. Hold your breath out for a count of three, then breathe in and relax. Repeat 1-3 times.

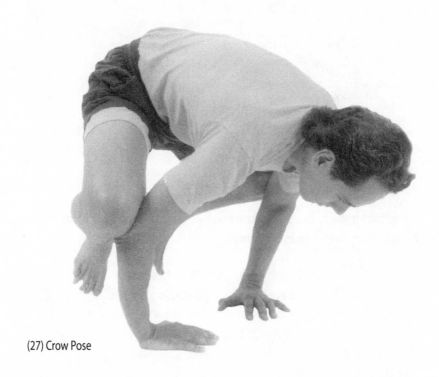

(27) Crow Pose

The flowing movements of this exercise recall the smooth movement of flowing water. When I asked my teacher Lakshmanjoo one day why Yogis love water so much, he said, "because it has no resistance." Imagine what it would be like if your mind felt no resistance to anything new, then imagine yourself in this exercise diving into new thought and new life rich with possibilities and with no limits.

HANDS AND KNEES STRETCH

Benefits: Limbers lower back; stretches chest muscles; improves circulation; loosens hip and knee joints.

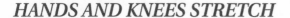

Starting from a hands-and-knees position, breathe in to a count of three as you lower your hips and arch your back, looking up and keeping your arms stiff (28). Hold for a count of three. Breathe out to a count of three as you sit back on your heels, bending forward with arms outstretched (29). Hold for a count of three. Continue the back-and-forth movement for three complete cycles.

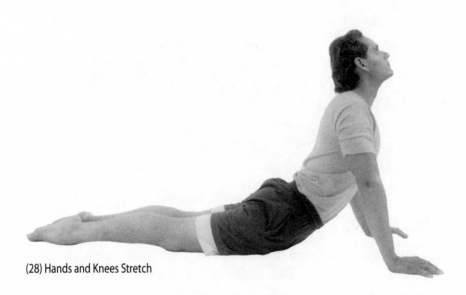

(28) Hands and Knees Stretch

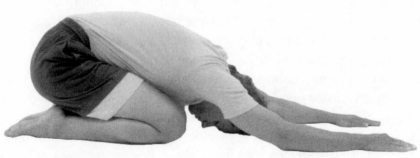

(29) Hands and Knees Stretch

When you practice Yoga regularly, you become flexible not only physically, but also emotionally. Being emotionally flexible means that you learn to be more tolerant of change and less judgmental of yourself and others. People who develop flexibility of mind and body are not troubled by the pain of resistance; they move with a silken grace and take on a youthful and beautiful appearance.

SPINE TWIST

Benefits: Improves digestion; limbers and tones entire spine; strengthens and limbers rib cage; relieves chronic constipation; helps relieve bladder, urinary tract, and prostate problems; improves circulation.

Sit up with both legs bent in front of you. Bend your left knee and lay it on the floor with your left foot under your right knee. Pick up your right foot and carry it across your left knee (30). Pull your left foot in close to your body.

Turn toward the right and bring your left arm over your right knee. With your left elbow, press your right knee back as far as it will go, then straighten your left arm and grasp the right big toe. If you can't reach your toe, grasp your ankle or knee instead. Bring your right hand close in to your body, fingers pointed in, and straighten the arm. Straighten your back, breathe in looking forward to a count of three, then breathe out to a count of three as you twist toward the right as far as you can (31). Look at a spot on the wall just above eye level. Hold your breath out for a count of three. Release, and repeat on the opposite side.

Variation: For a less-strenuous pose, keep your left leg outstretched (32), or practice the exercise in a chair (33). Seated on the edge of a straight chair, straighten your back and place your right hand on the outside of

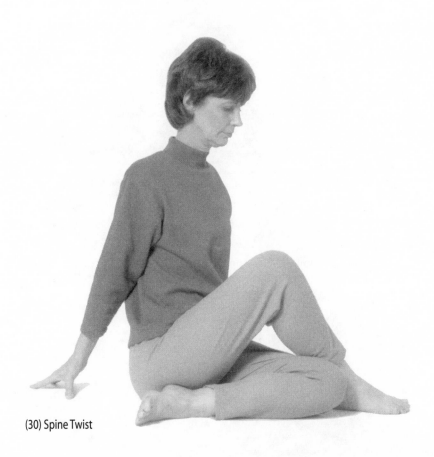

(30) Spine Twist

your left knee. Reach around the back of the chair with your left arm and hold firmly. Breathe in to a count of three with back straight, then breathe out to a count of three as you turn to face left, using your arms as leverage to twist a little further. Hold your breath out for a count of three, then breathe in to a count of three as you return to your starting position.

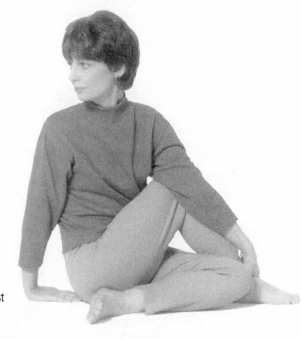

(31) Spine Twist

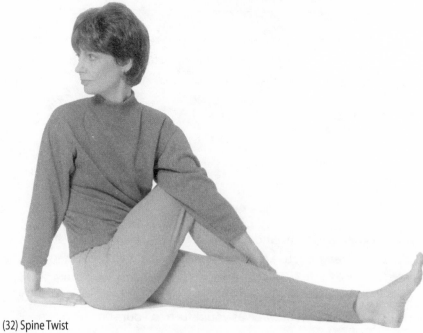

(32) Spine Twist

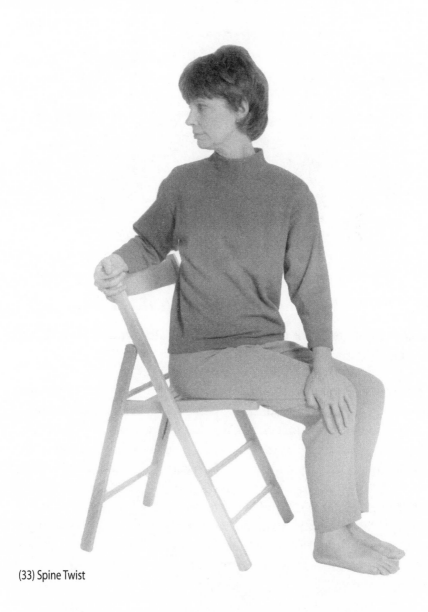

(33) Spine Twist

This Sun Pose is very effective in providing energy and health to the body. Practice it by visualizing the sun, just as you do with the Standing Sun Pose. As you become more proficient in this exercise, you will become aware of more graceful movements, and your posture will improve greatly. Good posture can help you look and feel better instantly. This exercise has long-lasting effects on the straightness and lengthening of the spine. I practiced this exercise every day in the early years of my Yoga practice, and I grew three inches after the age of 35!

SEATED SUN POSE (Paschimottanasan)

Benefits: Stretches back of legs; limbers and strengthens lower back; massages internal organs.

Bring both legs straight out in front of you and flex your toes. Sit straight, breathe out with arms at your sides, then breathe in to a count of three as you raise your arms in a wide circle to the sides (34) and overhead. Press your palms together, look up, and stretch from the rib cage (35). Visualize the sun. Hold your breath in for a count of three. Breathe out to a count of three as you bend forward, tucking your chin toward your chest. Grasp your ankles, bend your elbows, and pull your torso toward your legs (36). Remember to pull by bending your arms, not by pushing with your lower back. Hold your breath out for a count of three. If you are limber enough to reach your feet (and still bend your elbows), grasp your big toes as shown (37).

Release and breathe in to a count of three as you bring your arms out to the sides and over your head again. Stretch and look up as before, holding your breath in for a count of three. Breathe out to a count of three as you bring your arms back down to your sides. Repeat 3 times.

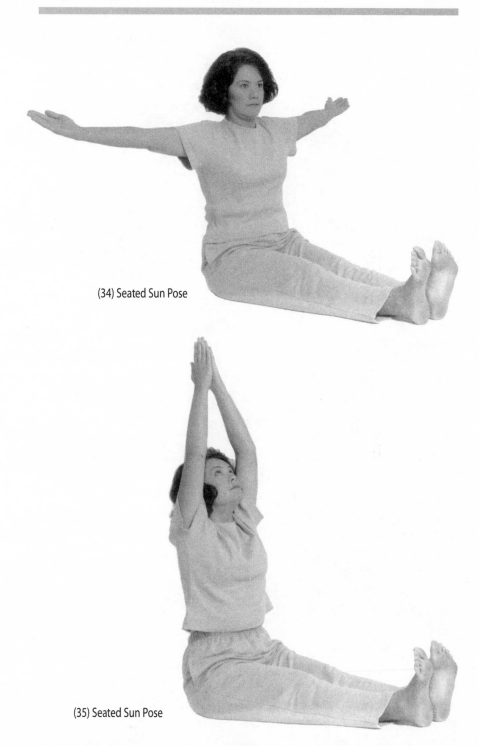

(34) Seated Sun Pose

(35) Seated Sun Pose

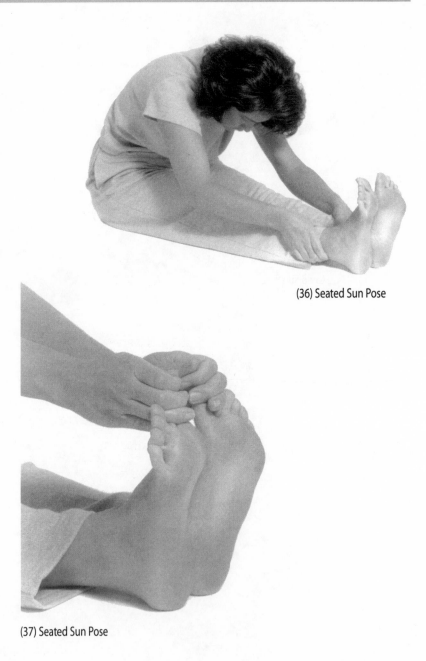

(36) Seated Sun Pose

(37) Seated Sun Pose

This exercise may also be done sitting up in bed with legs outstretched, back supported by the headboard.

Along with good posture, a graceful carriage is another sign of a person who feels self-confident, healthy, and strong. This exercise promotes an easy, graceful walk and good balance. As you breathe and move according to the instructions, visualize your back straightening, your hips aligning, and the oxygen circulating throughout your body, giving it renewed energy.

TORTOISE STRETCH (Kurmasan)

Benefits: Improves circulation to pelvic region through abdominal compression; stretches nerves and muscles in legs and ankles; limbers lower back; helps prevent prostate problems.

Separate your legs as far as possible and flex your toes. Straighten your back and breathe in to a count of three as you raise your arms in a wide circle to the sides and over your head (38). Hold for a count of three, then breathe out to a count of three as you bend forward, reaching down over one leg. Grasp your calf, ankle, or foot with both hands (39). If you can reach your toes easily, grasp the big toe with both hands as in the Seated Sun Pose (see p. 102). Hold your breath out for a count of three. Breathe in to a count of three as you raise your arms back over your head, hold for a count of three, then breathe out to a count of three as you lower your arms to your sides. Repeat 3 times to each side, then lean forward between your legs, grasp one leg or ankle with each hand and stretch forward as far as you can comfortably, relaxing your head and neck (40). Hold the position, breathing normally, for several seconds. Release and relax.

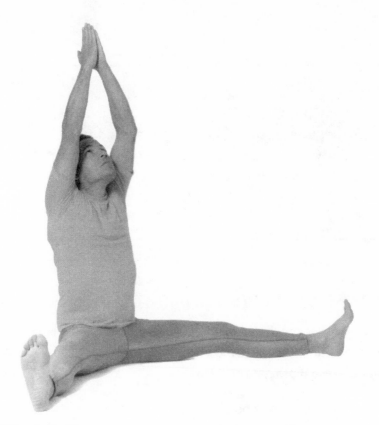

(38) Tortoise Stretch

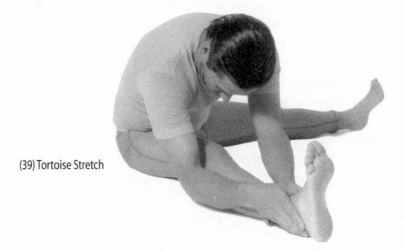

(39) Tortoise Stretch

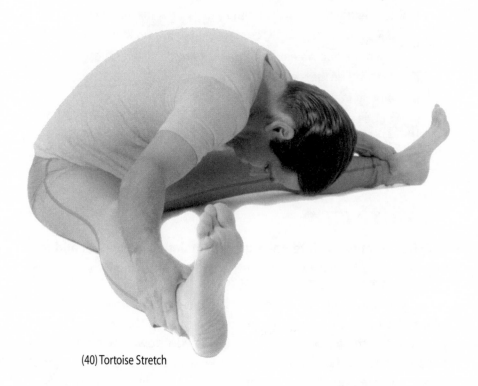

(40) Tortoise Stretch

This exercise will help you build a strong back, which is the cornerstone of Yoga practice and essential to health. A strong and limber spine can improve posture, respiration, and poise, and can help prevent the low-back pain and stiffness that too many people experience as they get older. Another way to strengthen your spine is simply to spend some time each day sitting without a back support, either in a straight chair or on the floor, in any comfortable position such as those described in the chapter on breathing (see p. 122). Adequate protein in your diet is also essential for a strong back, because protein builds muscle tissue. See Chapter 9 for more on how to be sure your diet includes adequate protein.

PELVIC TWIST

Benefits: Compresses internal organs, stimulating circulation and metabolism; reduces waistline; strengthens lower back and legs.

Lie on your back with your arms outstretched, palms down. Bend your knees and bring them up toward your chest (41). This is your starting position. Breathe in to a count of three as you slowly swing your legs toward the left as far as possible (keep knees bent). Hold for a count of three, then breathe out to a count of three as you lift your legs back to your starting position. Hold for a count of three, then breathe in to a count of three as you swing them to the opposite side. Hold for a count of three. Repeat twice more on each side, alternating.

Variation: If you have no back or neck problems, try this more challenging variation: When you swing your legs to the side, straighten them as they reach the floor (42), then bend them as they come back up to your starting position.

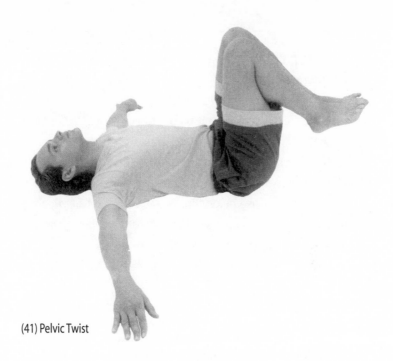

(41) Pelvic Twist

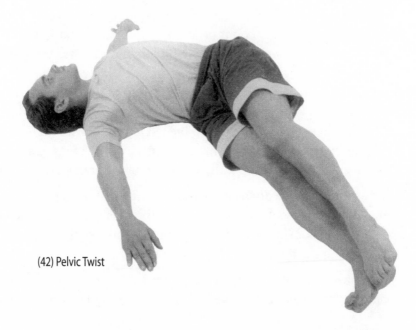

(42) Pelvic Twist

I used to pretend that this compression exercise was actually pumping illness and pain out of my body. I wanted to feel that I was able to help myself get well, and doing this made me feel better. I highly recommend that you observe your mental attitude while you practice all these exercises. Refuse a hopeless, sad thought while you practice. If you notice this type of thought slipping into your mind, replace it at once with positive, helpful conversation that will help lead you out of depression. Day by day you will benefit from this and help yourself to be the person you want to be.

KNEE SQUEEZE

Benefits: Improves digestion; limbers and relaxes lower back and hips; improves circulation in pelvic region; helps detoxify the body.

Lie on your back with arms overhead and legs together. Breathe out completely. Breathe in to a count of three as you bend your left knee and grasp it with both hands, bringing it in toward your chest, then squeeze your knee to your chest and lift your forehead up toward your knee (43). Hold your breath in for a count of three. Relax and breathe out to a count of three as you lower your head, arms, and leg down to the floor back to your starting position. Repeat with the left leg, then twice more on each side, alternating. (Note: If you have arthritis in your knees, grasp under the knee, around your upper thigh, instead of the knee itself.)

Rest a moment, then do the same movement with both legs at the same time. Hold your breath in for a count of three as you try to touch your forehead to your knees (44). Breathe out to a count of three as you relax back to your starting position. Repeat three times.

If you have difficulty getting on the floor, this exercise may be done in bed. You can also practice a variation of this exercise sitting in a sturdy

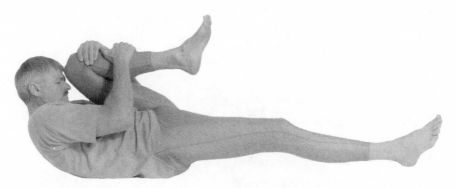

(43) Knee Squeeze

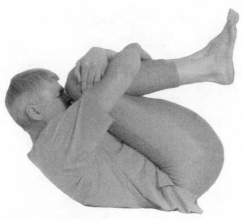

(44) Knee Squeeze

chair. Sit on the edge of the chair, breathe out, then breathe in to a count of three, lift one knee, wrap your arms around the knee and squeeze, holding your breath in for a count of three as you drop your forehead toward your knee (45). Then breathe out to a count of three as you release. Repeat 3 times with each leg, alternating.

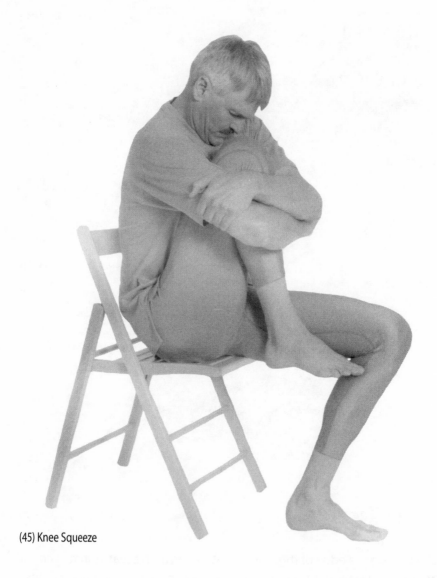

(45) Knee Squeeze

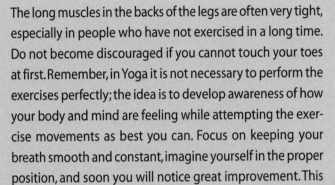

The long muscles in the backs of the legs are often very tight, especially in people who have not exercised in a long time. Do not become discouraged if you cannot touch your toes at first. Remember, in Yoga it is not necessary to perform the exercises perfectly; the idea is to develop awareness of how your body and mind are feeling while attempting the exercise movements as best you can. Focus on keeping your breath smooth and constant, imagine yourself in the proper position, and soon you will notice great improvement. This stretching movement protects against a humpback and poor posture by lengthening the spine.

ALTERNATE TOE TOUCH

Benefits: Tones and strengthens muscles in the legs, hips, and lower back; improves health of nervous system; improves respiration.

Lie on your back with arms overhead and legs together. Breathe out. Breathe in to a count of three as you lift your right arm and left leg and reach for your big toe (46). If you can, grasp the toe with your thumb and forefinger. (If you are very limber, you can reach around your big toe with your hand, as in the Seated Sun Pose, p. 102.) Hold your breath in for a count of three. Breathe out for a count of three as you lower the arm and leg. Another way to stretch into this position is to first bend the left knee, grasp the toe, and carefully straighten the leg as far as you can without strain. Repeat once on each side.

Variation: Lift arm and leg on the same side of the body, using the same breath pattern.

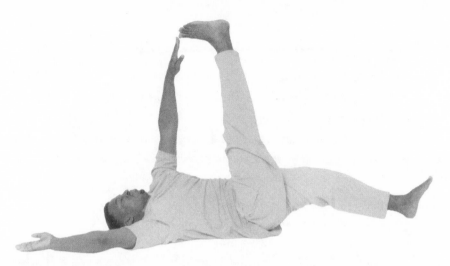

(46) Alternate Toe Touch

Yoga exercises were designed to benefit the functioning of all the systems of the body: muscular, circulatory, respiratory, and glandular. The shoulder stand is one of the most efficient and powerful Yoga exercises, affecting all the body's systems. The inverted position stimulates circulation and respiration, and holding your legs erect strengthens the large muscle groups. The pressure of holding yourself upright on your shoulders improves bone mass in the shoulders and spine. The glandular system is particularly targeted due to the increased pressure on the thyroid and parathyroid glands, located in the neck and head. When you perform the exercise correctly, your chin presses into your neck, putting pressure on the thyroid. The shoulder stand is one of the best exercises for weight loss because of this thyroid stimulation.

SHOULDER STAND *(Sarvangasan)*

Benefits: Stimulates thyroid and parathyroid glands; enhances function of all vital organs; improves circulation; relaxes nervous system; removes fatigue; improves bone mass in upper spine.

If you have known disk problems or chronic pain or stiffness in your neck or back, we suggest that you not do the full position; check with your doctor about trying the variation (photo 51) instead.

In a seated position with knees bent and arms around your knees (47), round your back and roll back and forth a few times, then roll back onto your shoulders, immediately supporting your back with your hands and keeping your knees bent and touching your forehead (48).

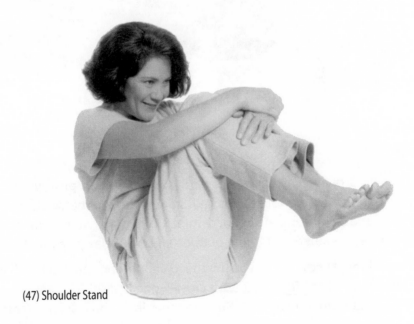

(47) Shoulder Stand

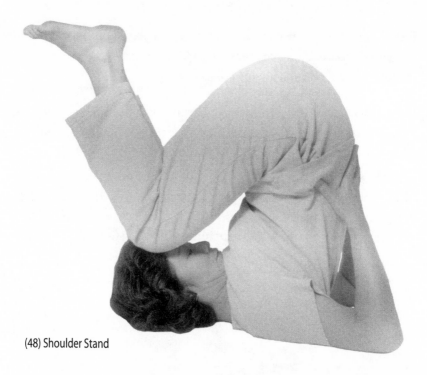

(48) Shoulder Stand

Slowly straighten your legs toward the ceiling and push your back straighter by using your hands (49). Stare at the spot between your big toes and breathe out to a count of three. Hold your breath out for a count of three. Breathe in to a count of three and then relax your breath.

Bend your knees back to your forehead, supporting your back with your hands, then roll forward into a cross-legged position, reaching your head and arms forward (50). Breathe naturally as you rest for at least ten seconds.

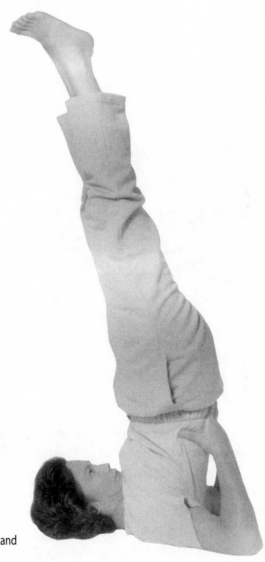

(49) Shoulder Stand

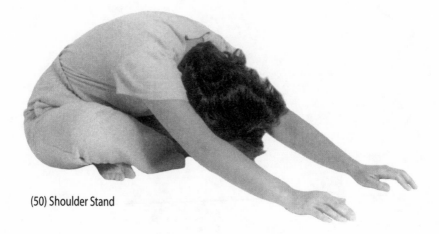

(50) Shoulder Stand

If you cannot do the full exercise, try this variation: Lie on your back with
your hips pressed against a bed or chair and feet braced against the edge
of the bed or chair. Breathe in completely. With arms at your sides, pressing down on the floor with your palms, breathe out to a count of three as
you push against the bed or chair edge with your feet, lifting your hips
and arching your back as much as possible without straining your neck
(51). Hold for a count of three, then breathe in to a count of three as you
relax back to your starting position. Repeat three times.

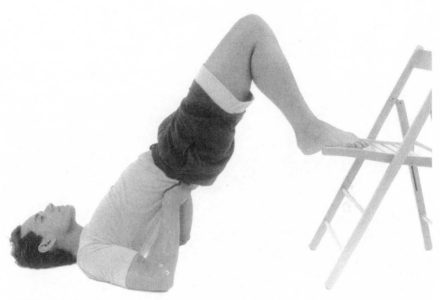

(51) Shoulder Stand

This is one of the Yoga exercises that stimulates the thyroid gland, located in the back of your throat. A healthy thyroid is responsible for proper metabolism and other vital functions. You will also appreciate the fact that this exercise tones muscles in the hips and thighs.

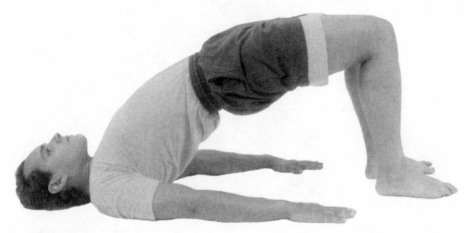

(52) Easy Bridge

EASY BRIDGE (Setau Badhasan)

Benefits: Improves functioning of thyroid and parathyroid and entire endocrine system; eases back pain and fatigue; increases circulation to head and face, improving complexion and eyesight; may help in management of hypertension.

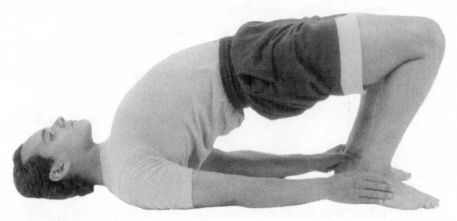

(53) Easy Bridge

Bend your knees and separate your legs and feet several inches; place your arms at your sides, palms down. Breathe in, then breathe out as you lift your hips, arching your back and tucking your chin into your chest (52). Hold your breath out for a moment. Repeat twice more.

Variation: If you are very limber, you can grasp your ankles with both hands (53).

This exercise is a powerful tool to help balance the nervous system pathways on both sides of your body. You will feel the effect from your forehead to your toes. You will know whether you have done the exercise correctly if all inner conversation stops.

COBRA POSE (Bhujangasan)

Benefits: Improves functioning of intestines; increases body heat; strengthens back muscles and limbers spinal column; increases overall body strength; strengthens eyesight.

Lie on your stomach. Bring your hands close in to your body under your armpits, with elbows raised, and your forehead to the floor (54). Breathe out. Breathe in to a count of three as you first curl your head back, then lift your chest off the floor, then your stomach, using your back muscles more than your arms. Keep your eyes focused between your eyebrows (55). Hold your breath in for a count of three.

Breathe out to a count of three as you curl down in reverse: stomach first, then chest, then head, bringing your forehead back to the floor. Repeat 3 times.

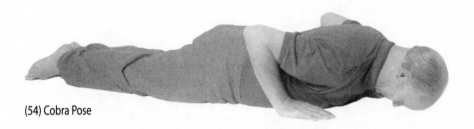

(54) Cobra Pose

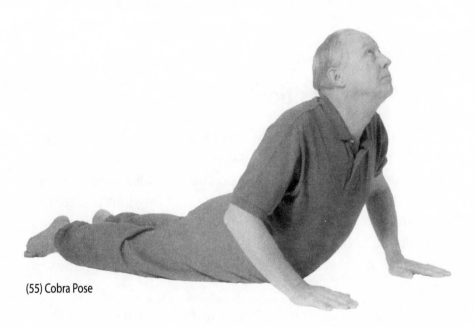

(55) Cobra Pose

Chapter 5

Yoga Breathing Techniques for Heart Health

Your Seated Position

Establishing a comfortable, erect seated position is essential. You have several options; be assured that you don't have to get into a complicated cross-legged position in order to benefit from breathing techniques! If you are quite stiff, or when you are first learning the technique, just sit on the edge of a straight chair, with your feet flat on the floor or toes tucked under slightly (56). Do not lean against the back of the chair. Rest your hands on your knees.

If your knees are fairly limber, you can try sitting on the floor, either kneeling or sitting cross-legged (57). If you sit cross-legged, be sure to use one or more firm cushions to raise your hips as

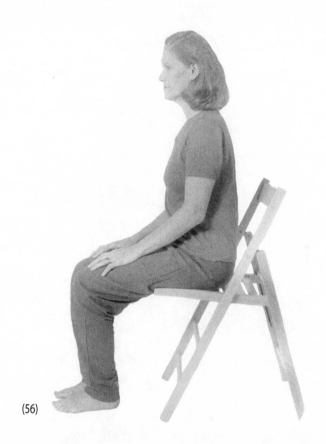

(56)

shown in the photo. This will keep your lower back and stomach from becoming tense, which usually results in slouching. In order for the breathing techniques to work, your back must remain straight and relaxed.

Always Breathe Through Your Nose

Always inhale and exhale through your nose — never your mouth. This is important in regulating the speed of your breath and improving your concentration. It helps to focus on the sound

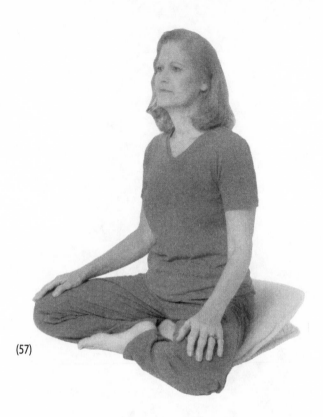

(57)

of your breath. If you close your throat slightly, you will hear a steamlike sound as you breathe in and out. Concentrating on this sound will help you keep your attention on your breath.

If one side of your nose is blocked, try this technique for opening it: If the right side is blocked, place your right fist in your left armpit and hold for a few minutes until the right side opens. Reverse the procedure to open the opposite side. Another method is to simply lie on your side for a few minutes: if the right nostril is blocked, lie on your left side. If neither of these techniques works, just do the best you can. Remember that although breathing through both nostrils equally is the ideal, you can still practice if your nose is partially blocked. The longer you practice Yoga, the more these passages will open.

When to Practice Breathing

When you are first starting to practice, do a few Complete Breath exercises at the beginning of your routine to help you get in the mood to practice and help you detach your mind from any cares or anxieties that you may be experiencing. Make the other breathing techniques in this section a part of your routine, preferably just before you lie down for meditation. You can also use breathing exercises — particularly the Complete Breath — any time of day to help calm stressful feelings you may be experiencing, to help manage fear or anxiety, or to change your thinking pattern. You can practice almost anywhere: lying in bed, in the car while waiting for a light to change (please do not practice while actively driving!), in a waiting room at the bank or doctor's office, or standing in line.

The Breathing Techniques

Belly Breath

Place your hands loosely on your belly below your navel. Breathe in through your nose and relax your belly as you imagine that you are filling your belly with air, expanding it and pushing your hands outward. This movement will help relax all your abdominal muscles and cause the diaphragm to drop to its fullest extent, allowing the air to reach the bottom section of your lungs. Breathe out now, through your nose, and slowly, consciously, contract your belly muscles, pushing in with your hands until all the air is out. Repeat several times. Do not hold your breath at any time. Remember: as you inhale the belly expands outward; as you exhale the belly contracts inward. Move just your abdomen, not your chest. Your shoulders and neck should stay relaxed.

Complete Breath

In the Complete Breath, the movement of the Belly Breath is extended up into your chest, where you expand the space between your ribs all the way up to your collarbone, where you draw air into the topmost sections of your lungs. Always breathe through your nose, and concentrate on the sound of the breath as described earlier.

Place your hands on your belly and breathe out, trying not to slouch forward. Tighten your belly muscles to get as much air out as possible. Now begin to breathe in from the bottom up, letting your belly muscles relax so the air appears to fill your belly.

Continue to breathe in and feel the air filling the center part of your chest, at the level of your lower ribs. Imagine the muscles between your ribs stretching so that your ribs expand in all directions, not just forward. Breathe in a little more and feel the air filling the very top sections of your lungs (58). Keep your abdomen expanded as you fill to the top. Do not hold your breath, but gently start to breathe out, slowly, from the top down. First relax your chest, then let your ribs contract, and finally tighten your belly and push the last of the air out (59). Do not hold your breath at the bottom of the cycle either. Repeat the Complete Breath three to ten times.

Depending on your current breath capacity, the complete cycle of the Complete Breath (one inhalation, one exhalation) may take 10 to 30 seconds. It is important to breathe in and out for

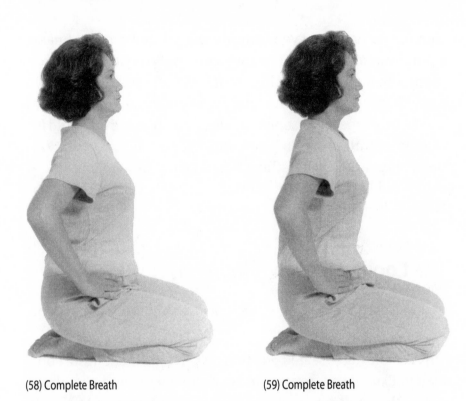

(58) Complete Breath   (59) Complete Breath

approximately the same length of time. Most of us naturally breathe out longer than we breathe in. In the Complete Breath you are counteracting that tendency and breathing more evenly.

Alternate Nostril Breath

The main purpose for this breathing technique is to balance the two sides of the body and the two bodies, the physical and spiritual.

In a comfortable seated position or in a chair, curl the first and second fingers of your right hand inward, holding them down with the fleshy part of your thumb. The third and fourth fingers should remain extended. Close your right nostril with your thumb (60), and breathe in through the left nostril only. Hold for a count of three, then close the left nostril with your third and fourth fingers (61), open the right, and breathe out, hold for a count of three, then in again, through the right nostril. Continue alternating by breathing out, then in, through one side at a time, holding for a count of three at each transition from inhalation to exhalation. Repeat 5-10 times.

The Cooling Breath *(Sitali)*

This technique has a cooling effect on the body; it also improves resistance to disease and enhances physical beauty.

In a comfortable seated position or in a chair, breathe out completely. Extend your tongue and curl the sides in (62). Breathe in slowly, then hold for a count of three. Exhale with mouth closed. Hold for a count of three. Make the inhalation and exhalation equal in length. Repeat 5-10 times.

Soft Bellows Breath *(Kapalabhati)*

This exercise tones and relaxes the muscles and nerves involved in respiration. It is an excellent preparatory technique for meditation because it focuses the mind very quickly. Its Sanskrit name literally means "shining skull," which refers to the power of this technique to stimulate the movement of energy through the body to the top of the head. In mythical language this implies that a lotus is opening at the top of the head.

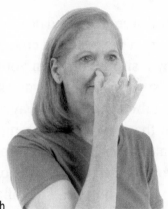

(60) Alternate Nostril Breath

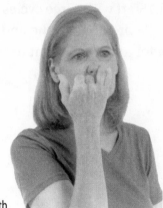

(61) Alternate Nostril Breath

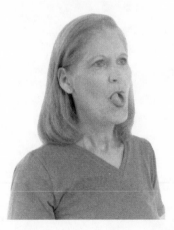

(62) Cooling Breath

Sit comfortably in a cross-legged position with your hips raised on cushions, or sit on the edge of a chair with feet tucked under slightly. You may rest one hand on your belly to monitor the movement, or rest your hands on your knees or thighs. In this exercise, you breathe in the same way as the Belly Breath but slightly faster so that you are breathing a little more strongly, using only the abdominal muscles. Breathe in for a count of three, then out for a count of three, without holding your breath either at the top or the bottom. The inhalation and exhalation should be equal in length. One cycle equals three inhalations and exhalations. Start with three cycles (nine breaths), and work up to 11 cycles (33 breaths). At the end of each cycle, relax your breath and rest for at least a count of three.

Chapter 6

Yoga Meditation for Heart Health

Your Meditation Position

In meditation you will be practicing "thinking nothing." To quiet your mind successfully, your physical body must be completely relaxed, and you cannot relax if you are straining to maintain an uncomfortable seated position. For this reason, we strongly suggest that you begin to learn meditation lying flat. That way, you can forget about your body while you focus on your thoughts and feelings. If your lower back feels tense, you can place a few pillows under your knees. Be careful to avoid pressure on the back of your neck. For this reason, it is best not to use a pillow; if you must have a pillow, it should be a small flat one.

If you are unable to lie on your back, you may sit in a chair as long as your back is straight — this is very important for meditation practice. Eventually, as you proceed in practice, you can try a comfortable seated position such as one of those described for the breathing exercises in Chapter 5 (see page 122).

Clothing and Equipment

Lie on the blanket or mat that you use for Yoga practice; if it is too short for your entire body, rest your head on it. Do not use a pillow under your head unless you have to, because it is important not to put pressure on the back of your neck. Wear your exercise clothes, and put on socks to keep your feet warm. Wrap your upper body with a shawl or blanket; your body temperature will drop as your body relaxes and your mind fills with silence, and you don't want to become chilled.

Protect Yourself from Disturbance

Ask family members not to interrupt you during your meditation time, and make sure pets are in another area. Turn off your telephone. Keep your practice space quiet and secure; sudden noises or intrusions can be quite shocking when you are completely relaxed and intensely quiet. Do not play music during any part of Yoga practice, because you want to experience your own thoughts and feelings free of outside influences. Silence is important.

Your Meditation Experience

Meditation is the key to bringing your two bodies, the physical and the emotional, together in harmony. If you practice a few minutes of meditation every day, along with a few exercises, you will soon begin to experience the satisfying power of operating as a whole person.

Classical Yoga meditation is not concentrating on your breath, or a sound, or anything else; it is simply no thought. One of the best ways to explain the meditation experience is that you simply try to stop talking to yourself. In the beginning, you may notice just a few seconds of quietness after you stop thinking one thought before another thought slips in. Meditation is a continuous process of increasing awareness. You start out in quietness, then before you know it your mind is full of plans, memories, anxieties, and other thoughts. Then you remember to stop talking to yourself, you are quiet for a while, and the whole process begins again. Try to remember what it feels like when you are not thinking. Eventually you will be able to recreate that feeling at will, and that will help you maintain the quiet feeling for longer periods of time.

Some people fall asleep when they first begin learning how to meditate. This is perfectly natural, and you will experience a very restful type of sleep. If you are practicing in the morning and are afraid that you will sleep too long, try not to use an alarm clock, because the loud noise will startle you and upset your system. Simply tell yourself mentally that you wish to meditate for a certain length of time and you will find that you naturally "wake up" after that time has passed. If you still need an aid to end meditation, try the alarm of a digital watch placed under a pillow so the sound is audible but not startling. I suggest that you begin by meditating for 10 minutes daily, and work up to 20 or 30 minutes if you wish.

Complete Relaxation Procedure

Lie on your back with your arms at your sides, palms up. Let your fingers curl naturally, and let your feet fall slightly outward (63). This is called the Corpse Pose. This complete relaxation procedure will take 5 to 10 minutes. The idea is to completely relax every bone, muscle, and nerve in your body so that you can forget about your body while you meditate. An audiocassette of the entire relaxation/meditation procedure is available from the American Yoga Association; see Resources.

Read over the following directions and then close your eyes and begin relaxing. You will be focusing your attention quietly on each part of your body, visualizing each part in turn without moving any part of your body except your breath. Simply tell yourself to relax each body part in your mind.

Start with your face. Gently and calmly bring all of your attention to your forehead. Feel all of the muscles in your forehead. Let them relax so they feel loose.

Become aware of your eyes. Are they tense and jumpy? The eyes are usually the most difficult body part to relax, so just let them loosen and float in the sockets. Let all tension and movement in the eyes stop. Move on to your lips, teeth, and all the muscles of the jaw, mouth, and throat. Let your tongue relax in your mouth, and say to yourself, "I don't have to speak for a few minutes." Feel all the skin on your face become loose. Let your scalp relax and imagine your ears drooping toward the floor. Your eyes may continue to jump around a little, but after regular practice you will be able to relax them more and more.

Now relax your shoulders, arms, and hands. Feel as if your arms were hollow. Let all the muscles of the shoulders settle loosely

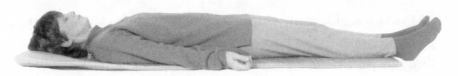

(63) Corpse Pose

on the floor. Move down into your elbow joints and imagine you can see and feel the bones. Relax and loosen them. Do the same with your forearms, wrists, and right into your hands and fingers, making them hollow and loose. Relax your fingers completely as though they were empty gloves lying on the floor.

Silently move your attention, like a tiny, warm relaxing beam of light, into your chest and, for a few moments, just observe the air moving in and out of your lungs. Feel your heart beating softly and rhythmically. Notice your belly rising and falling as you breathe. Do not try to speed up or slow down your breathing. Instead, just picture your lungs. Then take in a gentle breath of air, and, just as though you are sighing, let the breath out and relax your lungs. Take in another deep, gentle breath, sigh it out, and feel your heart relaxing also. Then let go of your breathing altogether, and relax all tension or effort in your breathing. Observe your belly and try to relax the squeezing effort as you breathe out. Each time you exhale, make your breath as relaxed as possible so that you are exerting almost no effort to breathe.

Now move your attention down into your legs, picturing them hollow, just as you did with your arms. Loosen and relax your thighs, hip sockets, and groin. Relax your knee joints and feel as though your lower legs are also hollow and empty, all the way into your toes. Imagine that your feet are empty — nothing inside, not even any bones. Feel your toenails relax and loosen.

Move up inside your empty feet, legs, and thighs, and bring your attention to the base of your spine. As you move upward through your waist area, relax any sign of tension so that your entire spine feels rubbery and loose. Feel your spine and all of its joints all the way up to the base of your skull. Spend a little extra time at the back of your neck. This common tension site needs extra attention. Imagine you can look right down inside your spinal column as though your spine were a rope dangling down into a dark well. Relax your spine so much that it feels as loose as that rope.

Next, concentrate on moving inside your head. Bring your attention back to your face to check whether or not your face is tense. Relax your eyes even more now, and let them float almost as though you can't feel them move at all.

Recheck the three main tension areas. 1) Is your breathing relaxed? 2) Are your eyes and facial muscles relaxed? 3) Is the back of your neck relaxed? Your body will eventually feel as if it were just an empty shell with no tension anywhere. The only movement will be your heart and your breathing, but they also will be very relaxed. Now relax the entire inside of your head. Feel your brain quietly settling inside your head with no effort or strain — just quiet and still.

Here is a summary of the relaxation steps:

1. *Relax your face and eyes.*

2. *Relax and empty your arms and hands.*

3. *Relax your lungs and heart.*

4. *Relax your belly and breathing.*

5. *Relax and empty your legs and feet, especially your thighs and knees.*

6. *Relax and loosen your back, shoulders, and neck.*

7. *Relax the inside of your head.*

8. *Recheck the three major tension areas: 1) your face and eyes; 2) your breathing; 3) the back of your neck.*

Meditation

Now you are ready to meditate. Start your meditation period by thinking of the sound "Om" (pronounced "ohm"). This word is a sound formula that has a specific effect on the mind when it is repeated or heard. "Om" is the oldest and most basic sound in classical Yoga. It has been said that if you could hear the subtle humming sound of the collective atomic structure of your own body and mind, that sound would most resemble the sound Om.

The Om sound of classical Yoga has been adopted and used in a religious way by nearly every religion of the Eastern world. However, in classical Yoga, the sound Om is used to center and focus the mind, and is not meant to indicate any particular religious concept or deity. Its purpose is to empty the mind except for the sound itself, leading finally to complete silence.

When you practice meditation, you will probably find that your experience of silence will be deeper and more refreshing if you repeat the sound "Om" to yourself several times at the beginning of your meditation session. Then simply stop talking to yourself in your mind. Try to stop all inner conversation. Don't force it; meditation is a process, not something that can be mastered overnight. Treat your daily meditation session like a game;

see how long you can be still before a thought interrupts you. Some days you will be able to be still for a long time; other days it will be difficult to stop talking to yourself or even stop thinking even for a second. Just keep trying every day and focus on the refreshing, quiet feeling that stays with you after your meditation session.

Eventually you will notice that this feeling will accompany you throughout your day. All you have to do is remember the feeling and it will be there. Many students tell me that their daily meditation period is as refreshing as taking a short nap. It is a tremendous help to concentration.

After Meditation

How you come out of meditation is as important as how you relax into it. If you get up too quickly, you may feel irritable or upset. When you open your eyes, before you start to move around, lie still for a few minutes longer thinking about the sensations, feelings, and thoughts that you experienced during your meditation period. Then increase your breathing a little to start reactivating your body and consciousness. At first, when you go to move your hands and arms, they may feel a little like wood since they've become so utterly relaxed. Make fists of your hands; then release them. Keeping your legs straight on the floor, flex your feet back toward your chin and then point them away. Do this a few times. Stretch your arms and legs like a cat does when it awakens from a nap. As you move toward your normal activities, you will feel refreshed, alert, and recharged with new energy and a clear mind.

Chapter 7

Yoga Fantasy Techniques for Heart Health

Whether you currently have coronary heart disease or are embarking on a program for prevention, the constant worry about it occupies a great part of your conscious and unconscious thoughts. It is always on your mind, and it affects all the decisions and relationships in your life. "Is the angina going to go away? Is it going to come back? Will I be able to do what I want to do today? Are obstructions forming in my arteries?"

Such constant discomfort erodes personal power. A loss of confidence accompanies all your activities, as well as loss of a healthy self-image. If you don't feel your best, you seldom find the courage to compete in daily life activity. It takes a brave person to live a full life in spite of underlying heart problems, and without becoming someone whose only conversation is complaint. Living with heart problems or the fear of contracting CHD may be a constant; how it affects you depends on the support that you are able to elicit from your inner body. The self-confidence that brings this about can come from the practice of Yoga, particularly through the use of fantasy.

Fantasy will help you adjust to a new way of experiencing your feelings about your health as you progress with our program. The physical body invents clever ways to keep its attitude from changing; you can counteract that tendency by practicing the ability to see yourself in a new body — one that is supple, relaxed, healthy, beautiful, and pain-free — each day in fantasy.

Many times, self-destructive attitudes are hidden in our vision of ourselves. Constant effort must be made to change your vision of yourself to what you want it to be, not a vision that portrays you as a victim. I have observed that most physical pain is due to one or the other of our bodies, the emotional/spiritual or the physical, acting with vengeance on the other. Imagine yourself looking into a mirror and saying "I hate my body for betraying me with these clogged arteries!" Neither the physical body nor the emotional body benefits from this scenario. What is needed is a new fantasy based on the idea of successful collaboration.

Often, in their zeal to begin getting results, people rush into a harsh discipline that upsets both bodies, setting the stage for vengeful reactions that often end in stalemate, or encouraging eating binges or even destructive escapes using alcohol, drugs, or nicotine. I suggest that you do not force a quick and ruthless change of attitude upon yourself. Start slowly, and create a gradual change of lifestyle — one that both your bodies will like. This allows your physical and emotional bodies to get used to the new routine, making it much more likely that you will continue. Most importantly, every day practice a fantasy vision of yourself as you wish to be. This is the support key to establishing that new vision as you continue to change your behavior.

How to Practice Fantasy Exercises

In the following pages I will teach you some easy Fantasy techniques to practice as part of your daily Yoga routine. The first time you practice a Fantasy exercise, set aside 10 to 15 minutes in a private place where you won't be disturbed. After you are familiar with the techniques, you can try practicing them while walking (see Chapter 8), or you can incorporate them into many other activities of daily life. An excellent time to practice Fantasy is just before you go to sleep at night. Note: Please do not practice Fantasy exercises while driving, operating dangerous machinery, or any other activity that requires your full attention for safety reasons. Consider your focus on safety at those times to be a practice of the Yogic ethic of Nonviolence toward yourself, and remember to practice your Fantasy exercises at another time.

Envisioning a Healthy Heart

Start by sitting or lying down in a comfortable position and closing your eyes. Take a few deep Complete Breaths and then let your breath return to normal. Let your entire body go limp and relaxed. In your mind, imagine your heart. It may help to first look at a picture in a medical textbook or encyclopedia to get an idea of what your heart and its arteries look like. Put every thought of illness out of your mind and picture your heart working perfectly. Imagine the happiness of your heart as you help it function with the many beneficial parts of your healthy heart program, including Yoga exercise, meditation, diet, exercise, and so on. Say to your heart, "I love you, heart. I am encouraging you in every way. I am so grateful for what you do for me." Continue talking to your heart in this way for as long as you like.

Now imagine all the parts of your heart and coronary arteries healthy and strong. Visualize the following changes:

• Blood flowing freely through your heart's arteries

• Sticky blood platelets letting go of each other and the walls of your arteries

• Blood clots dissolving

• Excess cholesterol and fats disappearing from the blood in your arteries

• Your arteries relaxing and expanding

• All fatty obstructions on your artery walls dissolving

• Your entire heart muscle suffused with new blood vessels bringing fresh oxygen

Complete the fantasy by picturing your whole self confident, poised, radiant with good health and strength — every desirable quality that you can think of. Hold that vision in your mind for as long as you can in silence. Then take another deep breath, let it out, and notice how you feel. I think you will feel some relief. Talk to yourself about how you feel, and remind yourself that you can recall that feeling whenever you need it or want it. Open your eyes and go about your day with new energy.

The "I Love You" Meditation Technique

This technique is one of the best ways I know to give yourself the confidence you need and want in order to keep up with your Yoga program for heart health. It is easy to do, and once you learn the technique, I urge you to use it throughout the day in different ways. For example, one of my students stands in front of the mirror every morning drying his hair. All the time his blow-dryer is on, he repeats "I love you" to his reflection in the mirror until his hair is dry. He says that this simple practice has changed his life.

This technique is a complement to, not a substitute for, daily meditation practice. (An audiocassette of this technique is available from the American Yoga Association; see Resources.) You will need to set aside about 15-20 minutes for this technique. Try it just before bed for a restful, refreshing sleep. Prepare yourself just as if you were going into meditation: lie on your back on your blanket, keep warm, and protect yourself from disturbances.

Start with what may seem a strange technique: Pump your arms and legs vigorously as if you were riding a bicycle, so that your whole body is moving. Laugh out loud and be as silly as you can imagine for about 30 seconds! This exercise will stimulate the brain chemicals that contribute to feelings of well-being. Then relax your body, settle into your meditation position, and let your breath relax.

Bring your attention to your forehead. Breathe in, saying "I love you" to yourself. Do the same as you breathe out. Repeat several times: breathe in "I love you" and breathe out "I love you." Breathe in and hold for a moment. Imagine the feeling "I love you" spreading throughout your brain in a beautiful, warm, wet, perfumed essence. Breathe out "I love you."

Relax completely. Let your breath relax. Hold that feeling. Then, for a few more minutes, continue saying "I love you" each time you breathe in and out. As you breathe in and hold your breath for a moment, think to yourself, "Whom do I love?" Breathe out and say "I love you." Breathe in and hold again; think: "Who loves me?" Now think to yourself: "My breath loves me." Breathe out. "My breath loves me." The breath is inside you. It loves you. Breathe in and think "I'm holding my breath — it loves me." Breathe out and think "I have released my breath — it still loves me." Take a deep breath, always through your nose. Breathe in: "My breath loves me." Breathe out: "My breath is gone now but it still loves me."

Relax completely. Visualize the inside of your head and your body. Think of the breath commingled with love. Oxygen is flowing through your arteries and heart and every part of you because you can't live without your breath. Visualize this loving breath inside your body. Are there any blocks keeping it from moving where it wants to go? Visualize this feeling of love and breath removing any kind of constriction, moving easily and sweetly throughout your body.

Bring the feeling to your forehead. Think "I love you — my breath is in my forehead." Relax your forehead. Now think of this feeling of love spreading to your eyes — you can almost see it! Relax your eyes and let the breath of love simply swim out into the rest of your face. Feel this breath of love in your nose, because it breathes for you. Every time you breathe in, breathe "I love you." Every time you breathe out, breathe "I love you." Let the breath of love flow freely so that your face melts with love. Let your mouth and throat relax, thinking "I love you" as you breathe.

Let your neck relax now so you have no constriction that will stop the breath from moving. Love comes in with your breath — relax. Love goes out with your breath — relax. Drop your collarbone toward the floor and say "I love you." Let the ends of your shoulders drop. Do the same with your arms; let them relax; feel that they are fully supported by this breath of love. Rest your arms in love. Relax your wrists. Let your hands be totally relaxed in love. You're vulnerable. You don't care. You can't lose love. Breath comes in and it goes out, and love is still there. Relax your fingers, letting them curl slightly, like a baby's hand when it is asleep.

Move your attention to your chest. Be aware that you are taking a breath into your heart: "I love you." Breathe it out with love. Breathe into your lungs: "I love you." Breathe out "I love you." Now relax your entire chest. Let your breath relax in love. Become aware that this breath is love. You're not making it happen; it's happening because it loves you.

Breathe in and think of your stomach. Breathe out and say "I love you" as you relax your stomach. Relax your abdomen, thinking: "I love you. I love you the way you are." Feel the breath of love move through your hip joint. Warm, liquid, lubricating, beautiful — perfectly balanced and poised. Say "I love you" to your hips and relax them. Let the large bones in the top of your legs sink toward the floor; you don't have to hold them up. You love them. They love you. You can't lose love. Relax your legs in love. Relax your knees and ankles and think "I love you." Think to your feet "I love you." Relax your feet.

Picture yourself just simply floating; completely supported on this breath, this love. Bring your attention up to the back of your hips and the base of your spine. Open it up like a flower. Say "I love you." Don't fight it. Let it flow easily, smooth and quiet. Relax the back of your shoulder blades. Let your back get soft. Love is supporting you. "I love you, back." The back of your neck relaxes. Think to yourself, "I love you. I love you." Then you reach your brain, your hair, all soft and supported, resting in love, in breath.

Breathe in and think love. Breathe out — love is still there. Think of your brain floating in a pool of this love. Make it totally quiet. Then simply say to yourself, "I love you." Bring your mind to your forehead and think nothing. Hold this feeling of quietness. If you feel any other thought coming in, make sure that it says "I love you." Transpose any thought to "I love you" and go back to thinking nothing. Think nothing as long as you can. Stop talking to yourself. Become silent internally.

Rest quietly like this for about 10 minutes, then slowly stretch, take a deep breath and let it out, and think about how you feel. Rest on your side or stomach for a few minutes enjoying the feeling before you get up. Move slowly back into your normal attitudes and lifestyle with a new vision of yourself.

During this exercise, it is important to note who is loving you. In reality, you are learning to love yourself. Regular practice of the "I love you" technique will open expression channels for your inner emotional body. It gives attention to the body that will replace the tension and stiffness that accompany pain. Every time you take something away from the physical body it must be offered a replacement for what it has lost or it will take vengeance on the emotional body. Similarly, if you deny expression to the emotional body, it will take vengeance on the physical. The goal is to find a happy balance where neither body fears the other. Fantasy is the best way to achieve this balance, and the "I Love You" technique is the basis for this practice of providing daily attention to the body in other ways than acknowledging suffering.

The Hall of Doors

This technique is very helpful for concentrating on a particular problem or concern. Using this technique, you can practice stressful interactions, face your fears about your heart and arteries, and deal with any difficulties you may encounter as you begin the necessary lifestyle changes to help heal your heart.

This fantasy exercise requires a concentrated period of about 5-10 minutes. Lie down on your back on your mat in the Corpse Pose with your arms at your sides, legs together, and eyes closed. Don't use a pillow behind your head. You can also do this exercise sitting in a chair as long as your back is straight. Stay warm. Completely relax your body as if you were about to meditate (see page 134).

Begin your fantasy exercise by bringing your inner attention to your forehead. Imagine that you are looking down a long hallway. There are several doors leading off this central hallway — some to the left, some to the right. Picture the hallway in every detail: the color of the walls, whether the floor is carpet, tile, or wood; the color and type of hardware on the doors; the lighting in the hallway — invent all these small details in your fantasy. Make it complete in your mind before you enter it.

Now before you walk down the hall, protect yourself by covering your entire body with armor. Imagine the most beautiful, heroic suit that you can, with all of the details, such as the color and weight of the armor, the type of helmet and gloves, the boots, and the fastenings. When your body is completely protected with armor, then create a beautiful sword of your own design and take it in your hand.

The reason for all this protection is that, in fantasy, you are exploring the unknown realm of your unconscious. Although everything in your mind is part of you, much of it will seem unfamiliar, and it might even feel a bit frightening at first. The conscious mind often feels anxiety about anything that is unknown; the symbolic protection of the armor and sword that you create in your mind lets you enter and observe your fantasy world without fear.

When you have a clear picture of your armor and sword, imagine yourself entering the hallway. Each door has a name written on it; for example, "My Heart and Arteries." Choose one of the doors, put your hand on the knob, and open it. Stand protected by your armor and sword, and simply observe what is in that room. Remember that you are not trying to create anything specific in the room; the idea is to experience something completely new — something that you have never experienced before. It will be a surprise.

Realize that you can step back and shut the door anytime you wish. I suggest that at first you try to observe for about a minute before leaving the room. When you decide to leave, shut the door, walk back down the hall, remove your armor, and observe yourself resting in the Corpse Pose. Give yourself plenty of time to change your orientation from the fantasy experience back to resting. Then, for a few minutes, think about what you have discovered.

The names on the various doors in your hallway can correspond to the concerns that are uppermost in your mind as you work with your healthy heart program. Some examples are angina, frustration, food, anxiety, relationships, work, and so on. Do not try to open all the doorways in one session; one at a time is enough! Try a new one each week.

Sometimes students tell me that they feel like quitting in frustration, saying that they never see anything when they open the doors in their fantasy. Usually I find that these people are afraid to try, which tells me that the obstacle confronting them is very difficult. If you find yourself in this position, simply continue with the fantasy exercise until you begin to enjoy some success. Probably you have never attempted to communicate with your unconscious mind before. If you continue to do the technique, eventually something will appear. I have never known a student who didn't eventually find something behind the door.

This technique will work best if you can practice it daily for at least a week. You will quickly experience great improvement in your concentration and your ability to deal with daily problems. Most of all, however, regular practice of this exercise allows the hidden, unseen experience of your inner body to show itself to you. It is no longer something that you just feel; it takes shape, and you are fully protected to face it and respond to it. When you have mastered the technique, you will find that you can use it as an immediate solution to whatever problems are hindering your progress in your Yoga program for heart health.

Chapter 8

Walking Contemplation for Heart Health

In any program for a healthy heart, regular exercise is important. Exercise burns calories, helping you to lose weight. Exercise also helps to reduce angina, by improving circulation through the coronary arteries. Regular exercise helps to reduce depression, anxiety, and insomnia; it feels good to both your physical and emotional bodies.

Exercise helps muscles grow, and your heart is the most important muscle in your body. With regular exercise, your heart increases in size as it increases its capacity to use oxygen. Its resting rate drops: blood flows through the coronary arteries between beats, so the slower the heart rate, the greater the blood flow to nourish your heart. Keeping your heart fit also increases its stroke volume, or the amount of blood that the heart pumps out with each beat. Exercise increases the levels of HDL in the

Benefits of Exercise

Encouraging reports from several recent studies suggest that walking can dramatically reduce the risk of CHD. In one study involving elderly men, risk of CHD declined 15% for every half-mile-per-day increase in walking distance. The participants reduced LDL, reduced the incidence and risk of blood clots, reduced the stickiness of blood platelets, and improved the flexibility of the artery walls.

Another study, from a decades-long project conducted by the Harvard School of Public Health, showed that the benefit of 30 minutes per day of moderate exercise, even when done in 15-minute segments, had long-lasting effects, reducing risk of CHD from 10% to 20%.

bloodstream and reduces the stickiness of platelets, so the blood is less likely to clot. Finally, exercise stimulates the growth of "collateral" arteries around the heart (as well as in other large muscle groups that are being used in exercise); collateral arteries are tiny supplemental blood vessels that grow and enlarge in response to increased demands for blood flow.

In this chapter, you will learn how to incorporate regular exercise into your daily life as part of your Yoga routine for heart health. If you can get into the habit of doing your Yoga routine every day, you will improve your concentration and the conditioning of your heart and arteries, and enjoy exercise more. It will not become boring.

You can practice this technique while walking, swimming, or riding a stationary bicycle. I have chosen to focus on these three forms of exercise because they are easy to do and, more importantly, they are not dangerous to do while your attention is elsewhere. They are low-impact — much easier on your joints than running or other high-impact sports. I do not recommend cycling on the street, simply because you will have to pay too much attention to traffic and other hazards to be able to concentrate fully on the technique. If you are an experienced exerciser used to running or jogging, you can try adapting this technique for use on a treadmill.

Bhairavi Mudra

The technique called Walking Contemplation is based on an ancient Yogic technique called *Bhairavi Mudra* (bye-RAH-vee MOO-dra). Both of my great teachers used this technique while walking in the mountains of Kashmir. Here is a rough translation of the ancient text that describes the technique:

> *Bhairavi mudra is a pose in which the eyes are open externally without blinking, but the attention is turned to the inner essential Self. Though the eyes are open, the aspirant sees nothing of the external world.*

This is a bit like meditating with your eyes open. Think of the "inner essential Self" as the feeling of stillness that you experience while meditating (see Chapter 6). While you are walking (or swimming or cycling), simply turn your mind inward and

The Ethic of Nonhoarding

The practice of Bhairavi Mudra will sharpen your awareness of the subtle aspects of hoarding. Whenever you name an object that you see — flowers, fence, etc. — you are, in a sense, owning that object. In Walking Contemplation, you are trying to reduce that outward reach of your mind in order to focus on the feeling of stillness. The experience of that stillness, where "names and forms" (*namarupa*, in Sanskrit) leave the mind, is one aspect of the ethical practice of Nonhoarding.

try to reexperience the feeling of stillness. Stop talking to yourself internally.

Try to turn all your senses inward as well. For instance, you see the roses in your neighbor's garden as you pass by. While practicing Walking Contemplation, you try not to name the flowers or let your thoughts turn to your own garden; you just experience the sensation of seeing the colors and shapes and move on as you feel stillness inside. You may hear birds singing, or other noises; try not to name the noise or look for it, but simply walk on with your attention turned to inner silence. In other words, try not to use language in the experience; language becomes judgmental.

You will find this to be a continual process. Just as in the concentrated meditation period that you do as part of your daily Yoga routine (see Chapter 6), you will find that sometimes it is easier to feel stillness than at other times. In the beginning you may be able to focus on stillness only for a few seconds at a time. Eventually, something that you see or hear or remember starts the thinking process — and inner talking — again. Whenever you notice yourself thinking about something else, gently bring your attention back to stillness. Don't force it, and try not to judge yourself. Look at it as a game that you are playing with yourself. See how long you can do it.

When I first began this practice, I tried it while walking through a department store and was overwhelmed by the seemingly infinite number of recognitions, categorizations, and even judgments that my brain was capable of producing. It was as if the huge number of objects surrounding me were all demanding a response from me, which was distracting and upsetting, even to the point of often becoming sick to my stomach. If you find that you are always tired after a shopping trip, perhaps you are experiencing this also, and you might find the technique of *Bhairavi Mudra* helpful. After long practice of this technique myself, I have found that the chaos of these earlier adventures is much reduced, and trips to the mall are a lot more peaceful.

If you find that it is too hard to focus on stillness at first, or if you just want a change of pace, you can substitute other subjects for contemplation. Here are a few suggestions:

Focus on Nonviolence, or some other ethic. Use your exercise time to consider how you can practice Nonviolence in yourself, such as stopping self-critical thoughts, counteracting feelings of helplessness, eating the right foods, and so on. (If you are interested in finding out more about Nonviolence and other ethics of Yoga, they are discussed at length in my book *Yoga of the Heart*; see Resources.)

In other sessions, focus on practicing Nonviolence toward others, such as a spouse, child, or co-worker; think about some ways in which you may have acted in a hurtful way toward the person, and mentally rehearse future interactions in which you respond nonviolently. Practice other ethical principles in the same way. Lakshmanjoo always reminded me to remember how to recognize Truth. He said, "Truth is sweet. It is always sweet. So you can always tell if you are speaking Truth."

Practice the "I Love You" technique. While you are exercising, practice the "I Love You" technique in your mind (see page 143), repeating the phrase on your breath and carrying it throughout your body just as if you were lying down.

Watch your breath. In the same way that you concentrate on stillness, concentrate on your breath. Do not change your breath; simply watch it. Listen to the sound of your breath as you walk. (See page 124 for more on the sound of your breath.) It helps to talk to your breath: Encourage it and praise it.

Your Exercise Program

Do you need a stress test before starting an exercise program? Most experts suggest it if you are over 40 with symptoms of coronary heart disease or with two or more risk factors (see Chapter 1). If you have special heart problems such as arrhythmia or murmurs, consult your doctor. At the very least, even younger people with a low risk of CHD should have a standard physical exam before starting a new exercise program. Please discuss this program with your doctor and decide together how to proceed.

Following are some tips to make the exercise portion of this technique more effective. Although these instructions focus primarily on walking, you can easily adapt them for swimming and cycling. I've added some particular recommendations for each form of exercise.

Start Gradually

The most common mistake people make in beginning a new exercise program is overdoing it, demanding too much of muscles that are not accustomed to being worked and creating stress by making too drastic a lifestyle change all at once. By gradually incorporating small increments of exercise time into your daily schedule, you will start looking forward to the feelings of relaxation and stress relief that exercise brings rather than seeing it as "one more thing I have to do today." If you start slowly, and gradually build up your exercise time, you will be more likely to enjoy it and keep it up as part of your new healthy lifestyle.

I find that people often overdo in the beginning, not out of naïve overenthusiasm but actually in order to defeat the effort. As I discussed in previous chapters, if the inner emotional body is not acknowledged and nourished, it will do everything it can to return the body to its previous state. The inner emotional body sabotages our plans with an initial euphoria which urges us to do more than we can sustain, making it more likely that we will overdo, "burn out," and eventually quit altogether. If you notice this tendency in yourself, try to restrain the impulse to do too much, and reassure your inner body with statements such as, "Little by little, I am changing my vision of myself. I will love the way I look and feel as I gradually create new enjoyable habits of diet and exercise." Another way to acknowledge your inner body

How to Take Your Pulse

Turn the hand of your nondominant hand palm up. Place the first two fingers of your other hand (do not use your thumb) on your wrist in line with the thumb so you can feel the pulsation. Count the number of pulsations in 15 seconds and multiply by four to get your heart rate. You can also measure your pulse by placing your fingers on your carotid artery, in your neck just to either side of the Adam's apple. There is no need to check your pulse frequently while exercising; occasional checks during your exercise session should be sufficient.

is through fantasy: Try the fantasy exercise of the Hall of Doors, picture your frightened inner body in one of the rooms, and then console it, "sweet-talk" it, in fantasy, and develop a closer communication with it.

The first two weeks. Whether you are very sedentary and unaccustomed to any exercise, or someone who is more active and wants to adopt a more regular fitness program, we recommend this single goal for the first two weeks: Get out the door and walk (or swim, or cycle) for a comfortable period of time four times each week. Practice taking your pulse (see sidebar) and calculating your target heart rate. Don't worry about time, mileage, or pacing; simply get used to practicing the contemplation exercise while you are exercising. It may be 5 minutes, it may be 20 minutes; just enjoy the benefits of taking care of yourself. Give your body a chance to enjoy a little exercise without taking the approach of a stern taskmaster.

Keep in mind that the goal is to develop a new lifestyle; a new way of looking at what is important to health and well-being each day. Although we recommend exercising four days per week in the beginning, set your goal on attaining at least five days of exercise per week eventually, and preferably seven days. If you start slowly and progress gradually, you will enjoy exercising so much that you won't want to miss a day!

Weeks three and four. Beginning in week three, add five minutes to your exercise time each week (never add more than five minutes per week). In week four, pick up the pace a little during your main exercise period, then add five minutes for cool down (see below).

Ongoing practice. Continue adding five minutes per week until you reach a total of 35 minutes (30 minutes briskly paced and vigorous activity, 5 minutes cool down) four or more days per week. See Resources for some excellent books on walking, cycling, and swimming if you'd like to refine your technique or add to your program.

In order to get the most from your exercise session, experts suggest levels of intensity, duration, and frequency.

Intensity, or the stress experienced by a hard-working heart, is measured by your heart rate. For the best fitness improvement in your heart, exercise hard enough to raise your heart rate into your "target zone," defined as 60% to 75% of your maximum heart rate. Determine your maximum heart rate by subtracting your age from 220. For instance, for a 40-year-old, the maximum heart rate would be 180 beats per minute, and so the target zone would be 60% to 75% of that, or 108 to 135 beats per minute. See sidebar, p. 157, for how to take your pulse. Work up slowly to

Incremental Exercise Works Too

You don't have to exercise all at once to reap the benefits of exercise. As long as the exercise is vigorous, you can achieve the same results in three 10-minute segments throughout the day as in 30 minutes of sustained exercise. You can also add even more exercise time to your day by doing such things as:

– parking at the far end of the lot and walking briskly into the store or work.

– taking the stairs instead of the elevator.

– walking the dog at a good pace.

Just remember that your total time spent in briskly paced activities each day should add up to at least 30 minutes (not counting cool-down time).

your target heart rate, so that you can easily practice the contemplation exercise while you are exercising at all stages.

Duration. After building up the duration of your exercise gradually over two to four weeks, each exercise session should last 20 to 60 minutes.

Frequency. As suggested earlier in this chapter, try to start exercising at least four days per week, with the ultimate goal of exercising six or seven days per week. Most people find that it is easier to keep on a regular schedule if you follow the same pattern each day.

Warning Signs

If you feel any of the following symptoms during or right after exercise, stop! You may be exercising too hard, too long, or too often. Consult your doctor before continuing.

- Chest pain (angina)
- Light-headedness or confusion
- Nausea or vomiting
- Crampy pain in leg
- Pallor or bluish skin tone
- Breathlessness that lasts longer than ten minutes
- Palpitations

Warm Up

Always begin your exercise session by walking slowly for a few minutes before you begin exercising more vigorously. If you are cycling or swimming, ride or swim for a few minutes at a leisurely pace; in swimming, use a stroke that you enjoy most. If you are walking or riding a stationary bicycle, you will know that you are warmed up when you just begin to break a sweat.

Your Main Exercise Session

Adding no more than five minutes per week, work up to 30 minutes of total vigorous exercise time at least four days per week, practicing the contemplation exercise each time. You should be walking (or riding, or swimming) hard enough so that you are breathing a little faster than usual, but not hard enough so you get winded.

Hints for walkers: Watch your posture: relax your shoulders, keep your chin down, and don't arch your lower back. Breathe through your nose at all times. Pumping your arms as you walk increases the aerobic benefit while building and toning muscles in the arms, shoulders, and upper and lower back. Bend elbows at a 90° angle, and loosely clench your fists. Move your arms straight forward and back, brushing the sides of your body. Though it may seem natural to let your arms cross toward the center of your body in the front, pumping straight forward and back requires more muscular control, is gentler on the shoulder joints, and helps to prevent low back pain.

Hints for swimmers: Note: swimming may not be suitable for people with coronary heart disease if using a pool that is much cooler or warmer than 80 to 84 degrees. The target heart rate range should be 10 to 12 beats lower than for walking or cycling.

Use a variety of strokes: crawl/freestyle, breaststroke, side-stroke, backstroke. If you get winded, stop and tread water for a minute or two, or move to the side of the pool and practice some kicks (but try to maintain your contemplation exercise). Most authorities recommend continuing to move in some way during a recovery period rather than stopping completely. As your lung capacity improves, you'll be able to swim for longer periods.

Hints for cyclists: Your knees take less stress when you spin at a low gear (turn the cranks quickly and easily) instead of pushing a high gear (turn cranks slowly and with great effort). The combination of lower gear and fast cadence allows your muscles to work most efficiently. A long, steady ride trains your metabolism to burn fat more readily. If you are just starting out, take the time to choose a bicycle that fits correctly, and wear proper gear so that you remain comfortable. Find a location in your home where you can practice your contemplation exercise while riding, without becoming distracted by other family members, the television or radio, and so on.

Cross Training

Experienced athletes use cross training to increase their fitness and prevent injury. In cross training, you alternate two or, at the most, three forms of exercise during the week. Doing just one form of exercise trains only one set of muscles, while cross training works on different sets of muscles. For instance, cycling exercises the lower body primarily, while swimming adds emphasis to the upper body. Swimming may not burn fat as quickly as walking because it is not a weight-bearing exercise; however, walking is harder on the joints, especially the knees, and can be more strenuous for some people, especially if you are extremely sedentary. Doing a small amount of two forms of exercise prevents injury by varying the work that your joints and muscles are required to do. And of course, preventing injury means no lost time from daily exercise. This technique also helps prevent boredom in your routine.

Wind Sprints (Interval Training)

A wind sprint is a short burst of higher intensity exercise in the middle of low-intensity exercise. For instance, after walking at your normal pace for 5 to 10 minutes, speed up to a much faster walk for 20 to 60 seconds, then slow back to your regular pace. Repeat every 5 to 10 minutes during your walking session. You can do the same while swimming or cycling. This short burst adds intensity to your exercise session without risking injury, and the brief extra work on your muscles means a more efficient fat-burning effect overall.

Cool Down

The cool-down period is as important as the warm-up. Walk, swim, or cycle at a slow pace for 5 to 10 minutes, then do a few stretches (on land) to lengthen the muscles that have contracted while you were exercising. If you don't stretch, your muscles will continue to contract and eventually start hurting due to the build-up of lactic acid. Here are some easy stretches that will work for either walking, swimming, or cycling:

Calf and Achilles' Tendon Stretches: (1) Stand facing a wall and rest your hands on the wall. Stand with back straight and abdominals in. Place right foot forward about six inches from the wall, and left foot back. Both heels remain flat on the floor, toes pointing forward. Ease your pelvis forward to feel the stretch in the main body of your left calf. Hold 10 to 15 seconds, then switch sides.

(2) Placing hands on the wall as before, stand with feet together about two feet away from the wall, toes forward and heels down. Keeping hips tucked in, gently bend knees until you feel the stretch in your lower calf and Achilles' tendon. Hold 10 to 15 seconds.

Toe Points and Ankle Circles: Holding on to a chair or bench for balance, straighten one leg in front of you and point your toes, then flex them. Repeat several times, then switch legs. Next, stretch one leg in front of you and rotate the ankle 5 to 10 times in each direction. Repeat with the other ankle.

Forward Bend: Stand with feet parallel, a few inches apart. Breathe in deeply, stretching your arms wide to the sides, then breathe out and bend forward, keeping your knees straight but not locked (if you have any lower back discomfort, you can bend your knees slightly). Let your upper body relax, especially your arms and head. Stay in the forward position for about 20 seconds, breathing normally. Then breathe in as you slowly straighten.

Heel Back: Holding on to a chair or bench for balance with your left hand, bend your right knee and grasp the toes of your right foot with your right hand. Pull the foot gently toward your body, stopping when you feel a pull in your thigh. Hold for about 20 seconds, breathing normally. Do this twice on each leg, alternating.

Shoulder Stretch: Reach straight up with one hand as if trying to touch the ceiling. Now reach up behind your head with the other hand and pull the elbow across above your head slowly. Stop as soon as you feel a gentle pull in the shoulder, armpit, or back. Hold for a count of 20, breathing normally, then slowly release and relax. Do this twice on each side, alternating.

Chapter 9

Essential Nutrients for a Healthy Heart

Heart disease, perhaps more than any other common ailment, is preventable and even reversible. One very important element in the change process is diet. In this and the following chapter, I will present very important information about how to change your diet. Up until now, it has been easy to explain our program and its rationale, as I have stressed how easy, gentle, and sweet the required changes are going to be, but now I have to get a little technical. You may even find these two chapters on diet too detailed to assimilate all at once. However, I want to stress the importance of the dietary principles described here.

Perhaps as you begin studying and practicing these dietary changes, you will want to slow down a little, read a few paragraphs every day, and allow time to absorb all this. I want to encourage you, no matter how difficult it may seem, to study a little of it every day. Even if it takes a few months to absorb this material and to put your new knowledge into practice, it will be well worth it.

Here are a few easy tips that you can begin with right away:

• Reduce saturated fat and cholesterol intake by eating less meat, poultry, fish, butter, and egg yolks; substitute soy and other plant-based protein sources. You will find a full discussion of soy protein starting on page 173 and a table of protein requirements on pages 176-177.

• Replace refined white four and sugar products with whole grain, reduced-sugar substitutes. Your goal is to eat six to eleven whole-grain servings per day and to reduce the amount of simple sugars; for example, replace white bread with whole-wheat bread and white rice with brown rice. Common serving sizes are one slice bread, and one-half cup rice, cooked or ready-to-eat cereal, or pasta.

• Make sure that you include five to nine servings of colorful fruits and vegetables every day. A serving is one cup raw leafy vegetables, one-half cup chopped or cooked fruit or vegetables, or one medium-sized fruit.

While you are studying these chapters, start with the above tips right away, perhaps by working with just one for the first week, then adding the second, and so forth. By doing this, be assured that you have already begun making the most important changes for a healthier heart, as these three suggestions are at the core of our diet program. You can add and refine the details later, at your own pace.

The Yoga Healthy Heart Diet

The diet in our program is quite different from the typical American diet, which is too high in saturated fat, animal protein, and refined carbohydrates. Our healthy heart diet plan is high in nutrients that protect the heart, and it will help you achieve and maintain your ideal weight. This plan depends upon plant-based protein sources, is rich in whole foods like fruits and vegetables, high in whole-grain complex carbohydrates, and low to very low in fats and cholesterol. The diet is rich in natural antioxidants, such as Vitamins C and E, beta-carotene, and selenium, to help protect the heart and facilitate the repair and healing process. I have also included a discussion of some nutritional supplements to ensure an abundance of proven heart-healthy nutrients.

The Yoga healthy heart diet is grounded in the idea of Nonviolence, the first and foremost of the ethical guidelines that are the basis of Yoga philosophy. When most people think about this ethic, they think of not harming others, but in Yoga practice your first duty is to not harm yourself. The strength of the partnership between your physical and spiritual bodies depends upon an attitude of help, not harm. Eating well is the most important act of kindness you can give to your physical body. Let's begin by examining some of the nutrients that help protect your heart.

The Role of Antioxidants

All cells in the body use oxygen to break down carbohydrates, fats, and proteins for energy. Among other byproducts, this oxidation process produces free radicals, unstable oxygen molecules that have lost one electron. Free radicals seek out and "steal" electrons from other molecules in the body. Among the substances that free radicals "attack" are the LDL cholesterol particles, leading to fatty streaks and plaque on the arterial walls.

As a way to limit the activity of free radicals and repair their damage, cells naturally produce a variety of antioxidants. As we age, however, our body's ability to produce its own antioxidants diminishes, which may be one reason CHD risk increases with age. A number of studies have shown a link between diets rich in antioxidants and a decrease in incidence of CHD as well as other diseases.

Some dietary antioxidants help reduce the risk of heart disease by preventing the free radicals from attacking LDL. Studies have focused on vitamin C, vitamin E, and beta-carotene, with some research on other antioxidants, including flavonoids, and trace elements such as selenium. Vitamin E and beta-carotene have been studied the most, because these two antioxidants are carried directly in the LDL particle. In most studies, participants simply added more antioxidant-rich foods to their diet. However, some studies have shown that the most effective reduction in heart disease risk has been obtained with levels of vitamin E that can be attained only through supplementation, not diet alone. I recommend vitamin E supplementation of 400 IU per day. If you are on anticoagulant therapy (such as aspirin or Coumadin), please consult your physician regarding vitamin E supplementation, as vitamin E may enhance anticoagulant effects. However, studies show that most people generally can well tolerate 400 IU of vitamin E.

Beta carotene, the precursor of vitamin A found in deeply colored fruits and vegetables, has not been proven to be absolutely safe as a supplement, so it is best to rely on diet. It is easy to add plenty of these foods throughout the day. At this time, no experts recommend additional supplementation of beta-carotene.

The findings regarding vitamin C are more inconclusive. Although vitamin C is not transported in the LDL particle, it has been shown to help preserve vitamin E in plasma, aiding in repairing the oxidative damage inflicted on vitamin E in the LDL particle. We recommend vitamin C supplementation of 500 mg twice daily. As for selenium, your daily multivitamin/mineral should include 200 mcg (micrograms) of this trace mineral.

Foods Rich in Antioxidants

Beta-carotene: dark green, yellow, and orange fruits and vegetables such as carrots, beets, oranges, and dark-green leafy vegetables. Note: light cooking, such as steaming or quickly sautéing, enhances the ability of your body to use the nutrients in these foods; overcooking, or boiling, decreases the content of most nutrients.

Vitamin C: Citrus fruits, berries, melons, tomatoes, potatoes, green peppers, and dark-green leafy vegetables. Note: cooking, storage, and processing depletes Vitamin C in foods.

Vitamin E: Vegetable and seed oils (soy, corn, extra-virgin olive, cottonseed, safflower, sunflower), nuts, sunflower seeds, wheat germ, and dark-green leafy vegetables.

Selenium: Nuts, egg yolks, and whole grains. Note: since egg yolks are extremely high in cholesterol, our low-cholesterol diet does not provide sufficient egg yolks to be a good source of any nutrients.

The B Vitamin–Homocysteine Connection

Several studies have shown a connection between high blood levels of homocysteine and an increased risk of heart disease. Homocysteine is an amino acid normally found in the body as a byproduct of protein metabolism. Although the link between elevated blood levels of homocysteine and CHD is not completely understood, researchers believe that too much homocysteine causes thickening and scarring in the arterial lining. This can lead to a build-up of cholesterol resulting in blood clots or clogging of the arteries.

Blood levels of homocysteine are influenced by genetics as well as dietary factors. The B vitamins folic acid (folate), B-6, and B-12 work together to help rid the body of homocysteine. Studies have found a link between low folate levels in the blood with high homocysteine levels and a greater risk of heart disease. A Canadian study of more than 5,000 people found that 25% of those studied who had the lowest folate levels were 69% more likely to die of a coronary problem than those 25% with the highest folate levels. Many people fall short of the minimum daily requirement for folic acid (200 micrograms/day). Some research suggests that most people should supplement with at least 400 micrograms of folate daily to maintain optimal blood levels, and most multivitamins include this amount.

As we age, our bodies become less efficient at storing B vitamins, which may be why many adults have low B-12 and folate levels. A balanced diet can usually provide enough sources of B-6 and B-12, although a recent survey of 3,000 men and women found a surprising 40% of all ages with blood levels of B-12 low enough for neurological signs of deficiency and high homocysteine levels to occur. Surprisingly, those who supplemented had higher levels of B-12 than those eating a diet richer in B-12.

Foods Rich in B-6, B-12, and Folate (Folic Acid)

Vitamin B-6 is found in eggs, soy, oats, whole wheat, peanuts, and bananas. Vitamin B-12 is found in dairy products, nutritional yeast, fortified soy milk, soy products, and some cereals (read the labels), in addition to high-fat-and-cholesterol-containing meat, poultry, and fish. Folate is found in citrus fruits, dark-green vegetables such as spinach (cooked) and broccoli (raw), cereals and other grain-based foods fortified with folic acid, and beans such as lentils and chick peas.

Phytochemicals

Phytochemicals (phyto is a Greek prefix meaning plant-based) are compounds found in all plant food sources: fruits, vegetables, whole grains, beans, nuts, and seeds. Many phytochemicals may have an effect on reducing the risk of cardiovascular disease, though we need a lot more information in order to be sure about the specific functions of different phytochemicals in the body, which ones are most effective in reducing risks of heart disease, and what quantities the body needs for maximum benefit. So far, studies have focused on three main categories of phytochemicals: sulfur compounds, flavonoids, and soy proteins, including isoflavones and phytoestrogens.

Sulfur Compounds

There is some evidence that foods in the allium family, especially onions, leeks, and garlic, are high in sulfur compounds that may help to lower cholesterol and reduce risk of atherosclerosis by decreasing formation of blood clots. A recent study

showed that consuming one-half clove of garlic per day may reduce cholesterol by about 9%. Because large quantities of garlic
can have adverse effects, such as allergic reactions and anemia,
don't go overboard; just eat normal food quantities of this plant
family regularly.

Flavonoids

Flavonoids, another form of antioxidants, are found in nuts
and citrus fruits, especially citrus pulp and the white of orange
rind. A study of 31,000 vegetarians showed that eating two
ounces of nuts five times per week reduced the risk of heart attack. Nuts also contain vitamin E, B vitamins, and minerals, all
of which contribute to a healthier heart. Most of the fat in nuts
is mono- or polyunsaturated, but nuts should be consumed in
moderation because of their higher total fat content. Depending on your daily calorie intake goals, including one to two
ounces of nuts in your diet most days in the week may be beneficial.

There are many different flavonoid compounds, and they contribute to improving cardiovascular health in a variety of ways.
Some flavonoids have antioxidant properties that protect the
body from oxidized LDL. Flavonoids may prevent smooth
muscle cells that line the arteries from clumping and contribut-
ing to plaque formation. They may also increase blood vessel
elasticity and resiliency, and increase concentrations of HDL.

Foods rich in flavonoids: Besides nuts and citrus fruits, other
sources of flavonoids that have been studied for their effects in
improving heart health are tea — particularly green tea — and
red wine. Moderate consumption of these beverages has been

shown to have a positive effect on reducing the risk of heart disease.

Soy Protein, Isoflavones, and Phytoestrogen

Soy protein, along with isoflavones, estrogenlike substances found primarily in soy products, is receiving considerable attention these days. Soy has been studied since the 1940s in animals. More recent human studies have examined the diets of Asian populations, who have a lower incidence of heart disease and diets high in soy products, to see if there might be a connection. In 1995, a review of studies involving over 1,000 subjects showed significant decreases in total and LDL cholesterol, and increases in beneficial HDL. The average consumption was 47 grams per day of soy protein — equivalent to slightly more than one pound of tofu or seven cups of soy milk!

The American Heart Association now recommends consumption of about half this amount of soy products daily, or 25 grams of soy protein, because the research is so compelling that soy helps reduce cholesterol levels. Also, soy has no cholesterol, is low in fat — especially saturated fat — so it is an excellent protein source and meat substitute. New fat-free or reduced-fat soy products are now available in supermarkets nationwide.

Studies have also focused specifically on the isoflavones or phytoestrogens in soy products and other plants. The heart benefits of soy are probably due in large measure to the isoflavones naturally occurring with the protein. Phytoestrogens are very similar to human estrogen, which helps reduce the risk of heart disease, especially in premenopausal women, as well as postmenopausal women on hormone-replacement therapy. In one study, consumption of 37 mg daily of isoflavones decreased total and LDL cholesterol by 8% in just nine weeks, in a group of people with high cholesterol. In general, studies show that soy and its derivatives have the greatest effect on those with higher initial levels of cholesterol. Some studies suggest that as little as one cup of soy milk or one-half cup of tofu gives a sufficient amount of isoflavones to be protective. Isoflavones and phytoestrogens seem to help the heart by:

• Blocking abnormal growth of smooth muscle cells in arteries that can lead to plaque formation.

• Increasing HDL levels.

• Providing antioxidant protection for LDL.

• Helping arteries relax to larger diameter (dilate).

• Decreasing plaque build-up that may lead to blood clots.

No one knows exactly how much of the isoflavones or phytoestrogen a person needs to consume to improve heart health, but a diet high in soy protein and other plant foods is very beneficial, in part because of its phytoestrogen content.

How to Incorporate Soy into Your Diet

The AHA recommends an intake of at least 25 grams of soy protein/day (roughly 2-3 servings/day) to guard against heart disease. This amount should provide 50 to 75 mg of isoflavones, more than enough to significantly decrease total and LDL cholesterol. One expert recommends anywhere from 8 to 30 grams of soy protein/day, depending upon your general health and the number of risk factors for heart disease. The table opposite shows the soy protein content of some readily available soy products:

Soy food	Serving size	Grams of soy protein
Soybeans	1/2 cup cooked	14 grams
Soy milk	1 cup	7 grams
Roasted soynuts	1/2 cup	34 grams
Soy flour	1/4 cup	8 grams
Tempeh	1/2 cup	16 grams
Textured soy protein	1/2 cup prepared	11 grams
Tofu	1/2 cup	10 grams

Here are some ways to increase soy protein in your diet:

• Use soy milk in place of cow's milk on cereal or as a beverage.

• Make a smoothie using soy milk, ice, and fresh fruit.

• Use textured soy protein (available in health food stores) or browned "tofu crumbles" instead of meat in sauces, casseroles, pastas, and stews. Another easy meat substitute is cubes of tofu (plain or rolled in herbs and spices) stir-fried in olive or canola oil until golden and slightly crispy.

• Substitute tofu for one-half the cheese in lasagna or quiche recipes.

• Substitute 1/4 cup soy flour for an equal measure of wheat flour in recipes such as muffins, pancakes, biscuits, and breads.

• Snack on roasted soynuts instead of pretzels or chips.

Protein

The average American diet supplies about twice as much protein as is needed, usually from meat, poultry, and fish sources
that are often very high in saturated fat and cholesterol. Your
body requires protein for building and repairing tissue throughout the body, and for hormone production. Protein seems to play
the primary role in the brain in reducing the hunger sensation,
so adequate protein will help reduce cravings and hunger pangs
— an important effect when you are trying to shed extra pounds
to help your heart. However, excess protein usually adds a lot of
unwanted calories and creates metabolic excess which the liver
and kidneys must process and excrete.

On a low-calorie diet, the body may "panic," believing that it
is starving. It then sets its metabolic rate lower in order to con-
serve energy, which prevents weight loss. To avoid this, be sure
that protein is adequate in your diet. Protein should constitute
about 15% of your caloric intake. If you follow the suggested diet
plan in Chapter 10 and obtain all the required servings of protein each day, you will be getting adequate protein.

How Much Protein Do You Need?

To use the following table, find your weight in pounds in
the left-hand column, and read across to find your protein
needs, in grams, in the column that best describes your activity level. Protein requirements vary according to age and
activity level as follows:

LOW — for most adults who are sedentary to moderately
active.

MODERATE — for active adults who regularly (daily) engage in fast-paced sports or other athletic training, or heavy manual labor, such as lifting, shoveling, etc.

HIGH — for a growing athlete, or an adult who is using weight training to build muscle mass.

Weight (in lbs)	Activity Level		
	Low	Moderate	High
100	40	50	75
110	44	55	83
120	48	60	90
130	52	65	98
140	56	70	105
150	60	75	113
160	64	80	120
170	68	85	128
180	72	90	135
190	76	95	143
200	80	100	150
210	84	105	158
220	88	110	165
230	92	115	173
240	96	120	180
250	100	125	188

The best low-fat protein sources are fat-free dairy products (milk, yogurt, and cottage cheese); fat-free "fake meats" made from soy products; and pure protein pills (amino acid tablets). Other low-fat sources of protein, such as peas, beans, and lentils, are high in protein, but also higher in calories from carbohydrates. Many whole grains contain a small amount of protein as well. If you eat meat, poultry, or fish, insist that it be as lean as possible. Invest in a small reference book that lists the nutrient content of various foods and count protein grams for a few days to be sure you are getting the required amount, using the table in the sidebar on page 177 as a guide. For example, if you are a 150-pound woman with a low activity level, you need about 60 grams of protein per day. Here is one example of how a menu of whole foods can easily supply you with more than this amount every day:

Breakfast: 1 cup fat-free milk (8 grams) on whole-grain cereal such as oatmeal (3)

Lunch: $^1/_4$ cup fat-free cottage cheese (8), sandwich made of mixed-grain bread (5) and two slices "fake meat" deli slices (18), 2/3 cup split-pea soup (6)

Dinner: spaghetti with tomato sauce (5) and tofu "meatballs" (7), fresh cooked greens (3) and cornbread (5)

(total protein grams: 68)

A few other common protein sources and their protein content are:

$^1/_2$ c dried beans	7
1 fat-free soy "hot dog"	11
1 c fat-free yogurt	13

1 c brown rice	5
1 T peanut butter	4
1 oz Swiss cheese	7
1 c nonfat milk	8
1 egg white	3.5
1 c low-fat (1%) buttermilk	8

Whole foods are preferred sources for nutrients, but sometimes every calorie counts if it is imperative that you lose weight. Pure protein tablets provide as much as 1.9 grams of high-grade natural dairy protein per tablet. Since the tablets are pure protein, this source is the most efficient at delivering the maximum amount of fat-free protein for the fewest number of calories. Plus, they are easily portable, so you can maintain your low-fat, low-calorie diet in restaurants and at work or play. If you use a pure source such as this, it is important to supplement your diet with iron and zinc as well as other vitamins and minerals that naturally accompany protein foods. (There is a fuller discussion of vitamin/mineral supplementation later in this chapter.) Important note: Never try to replace all food sources with amino acid pills, because this would be contrary to our whole-foods principle, and never use an amino acid source to exceed the required daily protein amounts.

I recommend that you obtain a significant proportion of your daily protein from plant sources such as soy products, whole grains, legumes, vegetables, seeds, and nuts. These foods contain both essential and nonessential amino acids, and they often combine to form the equivalent of even higher quality proteins. It is not necessary to eat complementary proteins at the same meal for this benefit. Soy protein by itself is the equal of animal proteins in terms of amino acid content. Many people believe that they need meat and other animal protein sources in order to get enough protein in their diet. This is not so. Plant proteins alone can provide enough as long as you get dietary protein from a variety of sources and eat enough calories to meet your energy needs — though not so many calories that you cannot maintain a reasonable weight.

Complex Carbohydrates

These are the best source of calories to fuel your muscles and brain, and form the foundation of our healthy heart diet. Complex carbohydrates come from whole foods such as fruits, vegetables, and grains; are naturally high in vitamins, minerals, and fiber; and are filling and lower in calories per volume than comparable processed and refined foods. I recommend getting about 55-75% of your daily calories from carbohydrate foods such as vegetables, peas and beans, fruits, and bread, pasta, and cereal. Whenever possible, use whole grain bakery products made with reduced amounts of total and saturated fats. These products are higher in fiber and B vitamins, other nutrients that are believed to help keep arteries healthy.

Some recent popular diet books say that eating carbohydrates prevents weight loss, and recommend replacing carbohydrates with high-fat, high-protein diets. This is dangerous advice for your heart, because blood fat and cholesterol levels will almost surely skyrocket. Further, if your body has to burn protein or fat for fuel, toxic byproducts (ketones) are formed. We do not recommend low-carbohydrate diets for these reasons.

Carbohydrates come in two forms, the first digestible, consisting mainly of complex starches and simpler sugars, and the second consisting of indigestible fiber, which has both water-soluble and insoluble components.

Digestible Carbohydrates

It is important to distinguish between complex and simple digestible carbohydrates. Some people must strictly limit their intake of simple carbohydrates, which can make blood fats rise. In people who are sensitive to carbohydrates, metabolism seems to instantly convert the blood sugar spike from rapid absorption of sugars into triglycerides, perhaps even raising cholesterol levels, too. There is no easy way to tell if you are this type of carbohydrate-sensitive person, or even how rare a condition it is. Instead, rely on a simple test: after three to six months on a low-fat diet, with no particular effort to radically reduce simple carbohydrates, check your blood triglyceride level. If it is higher than before, then the carbohydrates must be the cause of the elevation, so you must restrict them.

To be sure you are eating mostly complex carbohydrates, simply stick with whole grains! Another way to discriminate between carbohydrates is to refer to their "glycemic index," which is a measure of the carbohydrate's ability to raise your blood sugar in a given period of time: the higher the index, the faster the blood sugar rises. Not surprisingly, simple sugars like sucrose, dextrose, and fructose have the highest indexes, followed by alcohol and refined flours. Whole grains, even though they contain the same starches as the flour refined from them, are much lower on the glycemic scale because the fiber, which has not been stripped away by the milling process, slows down the absorp-

Glycemic Index of Some Common Foods

In order to set a base number, researchers fed subjects 50 grams of white bread and measured their blood glucose level. This was assigned the number 100. Other foods are rated in comparison to this standard.

White rice	83
Brown rice	79
Muffin	88
Whole-grain bread	48
All-bran cereal	60
Banana	77
Apple	54
Yogurt, low-fat, artificially sweetened	20
Milk, fat-free	46
Potato, baked	121
Peas, green	68

tion. Becoming aware of the glycemic index of different foods is especially important for diabetics, who must carefully monitor their blood sugar. The sidebar above shows some examples of the glycemic index of common foods.

Indigestible Carbohydrates

The indigestible or fibrous component is another good reason to concentrate on carbohydrates: High-carbohydrate foods such as fruits, vegetables, and whole grains are also high in fiber, which helps to lower cholesterol. Also, a high-fiber diet contributes to long-term cardiovascular health by lowering insulin levels. Finally, a high intake of fiber in the diet is also associated with lower weight.

The term "dietary fiber" refers to several materials in plants that the body cannot digest or absorb from the small intestine. Dietary fibers can be either water soluble or insoluble. Soluble fiber, which dissolves in boiling water, forms a gel-like substance that adheres to food particles. Fats bind to these encapsulated food particles and are eliminated from the body. Bacteria in the large intestine ferment about 75% of the dietary fiber that we eat. Some research has shown that the byproducts of this fermentation process may lower serum cholesterol.

While no one knows exactly how soluble fiber lowers cholesterol, numerous research studies have shown a link. In fact, experts now widely agree that soluble fiber helps to reduce risk of heart disease by lowering cholesterol. In January 1997, the Food and Drug Administration issued a statement that foods containing soluble fiber, such as those found in whole oats, may reduce the risk of heart disease when they are part of a diet low in saturated fats and cholesterol. The American Heart Association (AHA) also includes high soluble fiber intake as part of its overall dietary recommendations. I suggest that you try to consume an average of 30 grams of fiber every day, with at least 25 percent, or about 7.5 grams, in the form of soluble fiber. Most Americans consume less than half this amount, due to the shortage of whole foods in the diet. See the sidebar on page 185 for the fiber content of some common foods.

Recent research has established the value of lignin, a fiber found in whole grains and legumes; most vegetables also contain some plant lignin. Normal bacteria in the human digestive tract turn lignin into an antioxidant known as enterolactone. A Finnish study published in 1999 showed that men with high blood levels of enterolactone had three times less incidence of heart disease than men with low levels of the compound.

How to increase dietary fiber in your diet. Both types of fiber are important to health; foods richest in soluble fiber, which is the type believed to help reduce serum cholesterol, include oat bran, oatmeal, beans, peas, lentils, citrus fruits, strawberries, and pectin-rich fruits such as apples. Most other whole grains, for example wheat, rye, and rice, are composed primarily of insoluble fiber. The bran portion of the rice grain contains soluble fiber, and barley has some soluble fiber. Choose foods from all these groups to ensure a daily intake of a variety of dietary fiber.

Remember that not all oat, bran, and other whole grain bakery products (such as bran and carrot muffins) are low in fat, and some cereals do not contain much soluble fiber. Look for high-fiber cereals that contain at least three grams per serving, and always read the label to be sure you are getting a maximum amount of fiber in combination with low fat and cholesterol.

Some people avoid beans because they are bothered by gas from the bacterial fermentation in the intestines. If this is a problem for you, try discarding the soaking water and rinse beans before cooking to eliminate the indigestible sugars produced by the beans. You can also soak canned beans in water for one hour and discard the water. An over-the-counter enzyme product, widely available at drugstores, helps some people.

If you are unaccustomed to eating a substantial amount of high-fiber foods, increase your fiber intake gradually, and be sure to drink plenty of water (six to eight cups daily) to avoid constipation.

Sources of Dietary Fiber

Food	Amount	Soluble Fiber, g	Total Fiber, g
Legumes (cooked)			
Kidney beans	1/2 cup	2	7
Pinto beans	1/2 cup	2	7
Vegetables (cooked)			
Brussels sprouts	1/2 cup	2	4
Broccoli	1/2 cup	1	3
Spinach	1/2 cup	1	2
Fruits (raw)			
Apple	1 medium	1	4
Orange	1 medium	2	3
Grapefruit	1/2 med	1	2
Grapes	1 cup	0	1
Prunes	6 medium	3	8
Grains			
All-Bran cereal	1/2 cup	2	7
Oatmeal (dry)	1/3 cup	1	3
Oat bran (dry)	1/3 cup	2	4
Brown rice (cooked)	1/2 cup	0	5
Whole-wheat bread	2 slices	1	4
White bread	2 slices	0	1

Fats and Your Heart

Fats, or lipids, are a vitally important element of our diet that aids in the absorption of the fat-soluble vitamins (A, D, E, and K) and provides energy reserves, insulation, and protection for the body. You might be thinking, if fat is so important to health, why is it considered dangerous in the American diet?

The problem is in the types and quantity of fat that most Americans consume. Many health problems, such as obesity, diabetes, some forms of cancer and heart disease, are associated with excessive fat intake, particularly the saturated fats found in meat and dairy products (butterfat) as well as in fried and processed foods. A smaller proportion of saturated fats in the diet comes from a few plant sources, such as palm, palm kernel, and coconut oils, and cocoa butter. Some sources estimate that average Americans consume about 42% of their daily caloric intake from fat. To reduce the risk of heart disease by lowering blood levels of cholesterol and trigylcerides, we need to reduce our fat consumption into the more appropriate range of 10-30%.

There are three kinds of fats in the foods we eat: saturated, polyunsaturated, and monounsaturated fatty acids. Only saturated fats, along with dietary cholesterol, raise blood cholesterol. Most foods, animal and plant, contain all three types of fat, but in varying amounts and proportions. Cholesterol in the diet primarily comes from animal sources: meats, eggs (only the yolks), dairy (fat-free products have only very small amounts), fish, and poultry.

The body can use all three types of fats, but the recommended proportion of fats in your daily diet varies widely. For example, the American Heart Association recommends that total fat intake (saturated, monounsaturated, polyunsaturated) be no more than 30% of total calories for the average person. On the other hand, some experts in reversing heart disease recommend no more than 10% fats for those with moderate to severe CHD. Our three diet plans contain specific recommendations for the amount of fat in your diet based on your goals and risk factors.

Vegetable fats such as grain, seed, and nut oils tend to be less saturated and less harmful than animal fats such as butter and lard, but they are equally calorie-dense. Research has proven that polyunsaturated fats help the body get rid of newly formed cholesterol and reduce cholesterol deposits in artery walls. Monounsaturated fats also reduce blood cholesterol, but only when the overall diet is very low in saturated fat. In order to realize these risk-reducing benefits, it is imperative that you reduce your intake of all types of fat. If you are on a weight loss regimen, it is also very important to limit all fats.

Another reason to reduce fats in the diet has to do with a fatty acid called arachidonic acid. This substance aggravates inflammatory reactions at the site of arterial plaques. Animal fats such as butter, lard, and meat fat contain high amounts of this acid. Commonly used vegetable oils such as corn, sunflower, and safflower are easily converted to the same arachidonic acid. This is one reason I recommend using olive or canola oil instead of other vegetable oils. "Extra-virgin" olive oil has an additional benefit of providing some antioxidant protection.

Butter or Margarine?

To some, no table is completely set without butter, and few restaurants fail to deliver butter with the complimentary bread basket. Unfortunately, it is a food likely to increase plaque and clot formation, as it is rich in both saturated fat and cholesterol.

Margarine, on the other hand, is usually made from vegetable fat which contains no cholesterol.

Industry marketing efforts have presented margarine as an aid to all health problems, but this is not necessarily true. Brands vary widely in saturated and trans fat content due to full to partial hydrogenation; besides, margarine has the same calorie content as butter.

You must have heard our message by now: reduce fat! If you cannot face life without yellow spread on bread, limit its use as much as possible. And when you must have it, use the more liquid or tub margarines rather than stick forms, and avoid brands that use partially hydrogenated fats. Use naturally occurring, unhydrogenated oils such as canola or olive oil when possible, and try to avoid both hydrogenated and saturated fat.

Essential Fatty Acids

You may have heard about omega-3 fatty acids and their importance to heart health. The body requires two essential fatty acids (EFAs) for adequate biological function: linoleic acid (LA) and linolenic acid (LNA), collectively referred to as vitamin F. EFAs are polyunsaturated fats contained in plant oils, nuts, and seeds. They are commonly found together in food sources, although specific foods have higher concentrations of one EFA over another. The body generally requires more linolenic acid (omega-3) than linoleic acid (omega-6), in a ratio of about 2:1, but the vast proportion of EFAs in the diet consists of the omega-6 fats from common vegetable oils such as corn, safflower, and sunflower.

Alpha-linolenic acid (ALA), an omega-3 fatty acid, is also important to heart health. It is the precursor of two other omega-3 fatty acids (abbreviated as EPA and DHA), found in fish oils. Populations that consume large quantities of fish seem to have a lower incidence of heart disease. The omega-3 fatty acids play an important role as precursors of prostaglandin formation in the body. Prostaglandins are hormone-like substances that affect the inflammatory process and may help to reduce plaques in the arterial walls. They also reduce the risk of the formation of blood clots, help to lower cholesterol and triglyceride levels, and raise HDL cholesterol. Research results in the area of omega-3s are compelling enough for the American Heart Association to recommend increasing fish intake in the diet, although the AHA does not recommend supplementation with fish oil capsules, which apparently do not have a similar beneficial effect.

There are no vegetarian food sources of the omega-3s EPA and DHA, with the exception of red and brown algae. However, alpha-linolenic acid is metabolized by the body into EPA. Although this conversion is not 100% efficient, individuals who do not eat fish can substitute a teaspoon per day of plant seed oil, such as flaxseed, that contains ALA. ALA is also found in dark green leafy vegetables, pumpkin seeds, walnuts, and several beans, including soy, kidney, lima, navy, and great northern.

A word of caution regarding ALA supplementation: digestion of vegetable oils uses the same enzymes that are needed to convert ALA to EPA, so in order to maximize your body's use of ALA, you also need to decrease your consumption of vegetable oils. This is most easily done by substituting olive or canola oil for corn or other vegetable oils, which is consistent with obtaining the majority of your dietary fat from unsaturated sources.

Sources of Different Fats

Here are some examples of fats and oils in each group discussed in this chapter:

Saturated	Monounsaturated	Polyunsaturated
butter	olive oil	vegetable oils
cheese	olives	sesame
milk	canola oil	safflower
red meats	pecans	sunflower
poultry	peanuts	corn
coconut oil	cashews	soybean
	almonds	

Omega-6 (linoleic)	Omega-3 (alpha-linolenic)
sunflower	flaxseed
safflower	walnut
corn	anola
wheat germ	soybean
sesame	pumpkin

In summary, to follow a heart healthy diet with regard to fats, try to:

• Strictly limit saturated fats (all animal fats, including butter and lard; plus palm and coconut oils and cocoa butter, which are often found in baked goods and chocolate sweets).

• Also limit foods containing hydrogenated or partially hydrogenated fats, such as most margarines.

• Change your vegetable oil to extra-virgin olive oil and canola oil (especially for high-temperature cooking such as stir-frying).

• Add a small amount of flaxseed oil for omega-3 fatty acids (especially for low-temperature cooking and uncooked uses such as salad dressings); one or two teaspoons per day is enough to realize the benefit of this important fatty acid.

You'll find some specific suggestions for reducing the fats in your diet in the following chapter (see p. 212).

Supplements to Feed Your Heart

Food First!

Vitamin and mineral supplements cannot replace whole foods, which have hundreds of yet-to-be-discovered chemicals that may be important to health. Vitamin and mineral supplements have only a handful, so it is best to eat a wide variety of foods and to avoid chemical excesses and imbalances. Don't be one of the nine out of ten Americans who do not regularly eat the recommended number of daily servings of fruits and vegetables. Research has clearly linked a high intake of these foods rich in C, E, beta-carotene, and other antioxidants with a markedly reduced risk of CHD. The best strategy for optimal health and reducing your risk of chronic disease such as coronary heart disease, diabetes, and arthritis is to obtain adequate nutrients from a wide variety of foods.

Having said that, there are some instances in which supplementation may be a wise course. Primarily, if you have been eating the traditional American diet, you should consider yourself warned — it is deficient in essential vitamins, minerals, and fatty acids. Supplements help to restore tissue levels to normal levels. Also, if you are severely restricting calories in order to lose weight, vitamins and minerals may well be undersupplied.

Even a well-balanced diet can be lacking in adequate amounts if you restrict quantity and portion size. Generally, if you tend to skip meals, diet often, or eat meals high in sugar and fat, it would be reasonable for you to use supplements. Most of us eat as many as half of our meals in restaurants, which tends to limit our intake of nutritious foods. Finally, empty calories from junk foods are more and more prevalent as Americans consume even more fats and sugars with nutritional value stripped away.

Who Should Supplement?

Many experts believe that chronic health problems — CHD being perhaps preeminent — are related to a long-term nutritional imbalance: The body's ability to safely process cholesterol is overwhelmed by a diet too high in cholesterol and saturated fats. For CHD, it is imperative to focus on all aspects of diet affecting the body's ability to lower circulating levels of cholesterol and triglycerides, repair damaged arteries, and protect healthy artery tissue. Safe and effective nutritional supplements are an important part of this strategy.

As I mentioned previously, the older population most at risk for heart disease is also most likely to be overweight and restricting food intake to lose weight. Older people often have irregular eating habits and do not eat a well-balanced diet, even when not restricting calories. Loneliness, boredom, depression, lack of appetite, loss of taste and smell, and denture problems can all contribute to an older person not eating well. The bodies of older people do not absorb vitamins and minerals well.

Women have special needs throughout life, starting with calcium and vitamin D to prevent osteoporosis. Women of childbearing years usually do not get enough folic acid, which increases the risk of neurological birth defects and increases homocysteine levels damaging to the arteries. Doctors usually prescribe vitamin and mineral supplements for pregnant and lactating women, whose requirements are higher during this time.

Vegans (vegetarians who eat absolutely no animal products, including dairy and eggs) are unlikely to get adequate amounts of vitamins D, B-2, and B-12, or calcium, iron, and zinc, and should consider supplementation. Please see the vegan section in Chapter 10 (pages 225-227) for helpful information about how to make a vegan diet nutritionally sound, because a vegan diet is virtually guaranteed to be free of cholesterol and very low in saturated fat.

Best Food Sources — Vitamins

Here is a simple rule of thumb for getting your vitamin requirements from food: whole grains for B-complex, fruits and vegetables for vitamins A, C, and E. Citrus, bananas, cantaloupe, and dried fruits are all excellent; the vegetables with the highest vitamin content are always the most colorful ones. Dark green leafy vegetables such as spinach, colorful peppers, and all the members of the cabbage family such as broccoli, cauliflower, Brussels sprouts, and cabbage itself, along with carrots and winter squash, are all excellent sources.

All B-complex vitamins are included in whole-grain products except for B-12, which is found naturally only in milk, eggs, and meat from animal sources. Vegetarian or reduced-meat diets need a reliable source: Some easy sources are a multivitamin supplement, fortified breakfast cereals, and soy beverages. Eggs, to be used most sparingly, also supply most of the other B-complex vitamins, as do many fruits, vegetables, and meat. Vitamin D is added to milk and is formed on the skin by sunlight. Everyone should take a supplement with 400 mcg of folic acid, and our recommended multivitamins include it.

Best Food Sources — Minerals

Iron is found in high amounts in beef and pork (high in saturated fat and cholesterol too) and in moderate amounts in prunes, apricots, spinach, beans, tofu, blackstrap molasses, nutritional yeast, and wheat germ. However, all sources are dwarfed by the iron content of fortified cereals. For example, a serving of Total brand cereal contains 18 mg of iron, which is 100% of the recommended daily intake. Younger people, especially premenopausal women, need the full amount of iron, but older men and women probably only need 10 mg or less daily. Vegetarians need to be sure to include these iron-rich foods and to use a multivitamin/mineral supplement with iron. However, give some thought to the possibility of getting too much iron; it is a powerful oxidizer that can damage vitamin E, and possibly even oxidize LDL cholesterol.

Zinc is needed for growth and development, but is much more difficult to obtain, with only beef, pork, and shellfish being good sources. Wheat germ, garbanzo beans, and lentils are the best of the rest, but in order to get the recommended 15 mg, you would need to eat nearly 1 $^1/_2$ cups of wheat germ, for instance. A mineral supplement supplying the recommended amount of zinc seems to make good sense, and again, most multivitamin/mineral supplements include the recommended amount of 15 mg.

Calcium is highest in dairy foods — milk, yogurt, and cheese — and it is a good idea to include plenty of fat-free varieties in your diet. Other good sources include tofu (if processed with calcium sulfate) and dark green leafy vegetables (spinach, turnip greens, kale, etc.). Vegetarians absorb more calcium from foods, perhaps due to the lower fat levels in the gut. Unless you commit to eating at least four servings per day of high-calcium nonfat dairy foods (1 serving = 1 cup milk, 1 cup yogurt, 1 oz hard cheese), a calcium supplement should be used to replace each missing high-calcium serving. Calcium supplements should usually total 900 - 1,000 mg (three 300 mg tablets or two 500 mg tablets daily) for older people, since absorption decreases as we age.

Magnesium is an important part of calcium metabolism, affecting nerves, muscles in artery walls, and also reducing the risk of diabetes. Many studies indicate that Americans get too little. Whole grains and beans are the best sources, especially if they were grown in magnesium-rich soils. I take a calcium supplement that includes magnesium (about 1:3 or 1:2 magnesium-to-calcium ratio) for convenience, as the amount of magnesium in most multivitamin/mineral supplements is inadequate and the magnesium content of the soil my food is grown in is unknown.

Trace minerals are difficult to evaluate and should be sufficient in the diet, provided unrefined foods such as whole grains and fresh fruits and vegetables provide the majority of calories. The single exception is selenium. Add 200 mcg (micrograms, not milligrams) selenium to your supplement list for protection from prostate, lung, and colon cancers as well as antioxidant protection for your arteries. Most multivitamin/mineral supplements contain this amount.

Dietary Supplements and Heart Disease

Start with a good multivitamin/mineral supplement. This should be boosted with higher levels of several vitamins and minerals to help protect your arteries and perhaps even allow for some repair and rebuilding of damaged artery tissue. As I discussed previously in this chapter, antioxidants help to prevent free radicals from "attacking" LDL particles. These vitamins and minerals are also some of the key players in the artery repair processes. Wouldn't you prefer that minute injury to the walls of your heart's arteries be repaired before turning into fatty lesions and plaque? The vitamins A, E, and C are the principal antioxidants, so it would be smart to increase them to higher levels.

There are a host of other natural antioxidants in the news (lutein, beta-cryptoxanthine, flavonoids, lycopene, etc). All of them — and countless others as yet undiscovered by marketers — are available in plant foods, especially deeply colored fruits and vegetables. You must make sure that you include at least five to nine servings of these in your diet every day. All good-quality multivitamin/mineral supplements contain 5,000 IU of vitamin A. Vitamin C needs to be supplied up to 500 to 1,000 mg daily in order to saturate all the tissues. More than this is simply excreted. The best plan is to take 500 mg twice daily. Multivitamins usually contain only a small fraction of this amount. Vitamin E benefits seem to increase with daily amounts in capsule form up to 400 IU, and again, more isn't more. Multivitamins usually contain 30 to 60 IU. Calcium, magnesium, and vitamin D are all critical for bone health and often need to be supplemented: 1,000 to 1,200 mg calcium daily (300 mg three times daily is best) from citrate, and one-third to one-half that for magnesium. Vitamin D is included in most multivitamins and added to many dairy products.

Supplement Quality and Dosages

I usually go to large retailers where the price is lowest: Wal-Mart or Kmart, for example. The vitamin and mineral compounds in all supplements are manufactured by a small group of multinational corporations such as ADM, and "natural" vitamins are no better in quality. Many supplements include additives such as herbs and enzymes, but they contain these elements in such tiny amounts that they can do you no real good. The only quality issues for supplements are (a) nutrient content (does the tablet contain the labeled amount?), (2) whether the tablet will dissolve properly, and (3) purity. Although there are no federal standards for vitamins, you can help ensure quality by looking for the letters "USP" on the bottle, which indicates voluntary compliance with U. S. Pharmacopoeia, and by sticking to major brands; "store" brands are usually good bargains.

I usually take vitamin/mineral supplements after a meal for better absorption, and I take vitamin E and calcium at a different time of day than the basic multivitamin that includes iron. Calcium interferes with iron absorption, and iron may rapidly oxidize the vitamin E. Some experts suggest not taking vitamins and minerals at the same time as any prescription medications, so allow a few hours between to reduce the risk of interference. The basic multivitamin/mineral can cost as little as 10 cents or less per day, or as high as 50 cents or even higher for designer brands, though, as I mentioned earlier, there is no noticeable advantage to buying the higher priced brands.

Here are three steps to be sure you are getting an adequate amount of essential vitamins and minerals.

1. The best choice is to eat moderate amounts of a wide variety of foods prepared in such a way as to preserve the naturally occurring vitamins and minerals. The most nutritious foods are fat-free dairy products; deeply colored fruits and vegetables such as carrots, spinach, apricots, mangos, winter squash, and tomatoes; whole-grain bread and cereal products; and good protein sources such as soy-based meat substitutes, dried beans and peas, and, if you eat meat, the leanest possible cuts of meat, poultry, and fish. If some of the choices mentioned here don't sound appetizing to you, do some research and find some nutritious alternatives that you do like. It's important to eat food that you enjoy. This type of diet supplies a vast range of naturally occurring vitamins, minerals, and other compounds that science is just now learning about, such as flavonoids and phytoestrogens, that are not included in any supplement tablet. Fruits and vegetables can be eaten raw, steamed, or quickly sautéed to preserve nutrients; frying, boiling, and baking tend to reduce nutrient value. The nutrients in meat products are pretty much immune to such destruction, and grains usually must be boiled or baked for digestibility.

2. After you have fully established your new, more wholesome diet, consider taking a complete multivitamin/mineral supplement daily. Look for those that provide at least 100% of the daily value for A (often in the form of beta-carotene), B-1, B-2, niacin, B-6, B-12, C, D, E, and folic acid. Limit beta carotene to no more than 15,000 IU, iron to 10 mg, phosphorous to 100 mg, and B-6 to 200 mg. The supplement should also provide at least 25 mcg of vitamin K, 120 mcg of chromium, 100 mg magnesium, 2 mg copper, and 15 mg zinc. Iron requirements vary with gender and

age: Women under 50 need 8 to 18 mg of iron, men under 50 need under 10 mg, and men and women over 50 need no more than 10 mg iron. Everyone over 50 needs at least 24 mcg of B-12, because of generally poor absorption in older bodies. Everyone should have plenty of the antioxidant selenium, so make sure there is at least 200 mcg included.

A comprehensive multivitamin/mineral is a simple and relatively inexpensive choice. As I discussed earlier, you do not need to spend a lot of money on a supplement; the cheapest "store" brands are often as well-balanced and effective as the more expensive brands. When I was eliminating artificial colors from my diet to relieve symptoms of rheumatoid arthritis, I learned to buy uncolored and unflavored brands, or I rinsed the outer colored coating off, leaving the hard white shell on the tablets, before swallowing. Following are a few brand recommendations:

For Women — Centrum, Dr. Art Ulene Nutrition Boost Formula for Men & Women, Kroger Complete Extra, OneSource, Rite Aid Whole Source, Safeway Select Omnisource, Spring Valley Advantage, Summit Complete, Twinlab Dualtabs, Walgreens Ultra Choice, YourLife Super Multi-Vitamin.

For Men — Dr. Art Ulene Nutrition Boost Formula for Men & Women, Eckerd Daily Impact Senior, Rite Aid Whole Source Mature Adult, Safeway Select Omnisource Senior, Shaklee Vita-Lea without iron, Twinlab Dualtabs, YourLife Super Multi-vitamin.

For Older Men and Women (Over 50) — Dr. Art Ulene Nutrition Boost Formula for Men & Women, Eckerd Daily Impact Senior, Rite Aid Whole Source Mature Adult, Safeway Select Omnisource Senior, Twinlab Dualtabs. (Brand recommendations adapted from *Nutrition Action Healthletter* [see Resources], April 2000 issue.) At the time of publication, all of these selections, except for the Shaklee and Twinlab products, cost less than $5 for a month's supply.

3. Boost the potency of the multivitamin/mineral supplement you have chosen. As I mentioned previously, it is often useful to add more calcium, magnesium, vitamin C, and vitamin E to the daily multi described above. These nutrients are usually undersupplied in a multivitamin/mineral supplement, and they are vital for healing and prevention. Beta-carotene is richly supplied in the colorful variety of fruits and vegetables. If you eat the prescribed servings per day, you will have more than enough. If you short-change yourself foodwise, add 10,000 to 15,000 IU beta-carotene to your daily supplement.

With the above exceptions in mind, it is a good idea to limit your intake of vitamins and minerals to no more than 150% of the RDA, as large amounts of some vitamins and minerals can be toxic (especially vitamins A, D, and niacin, and the minerals selenium, iron, and zinc). The following table suggests how to take supplements throughout the day for best absorption.

Healthy Heart Supplements

Vitamins & minerals

Breakfast

> *Multivitamin/mineral*
>
> *B-complex*
>
> *500 mg Vitamin C*
>
> *1 teaspoon flaxseed oil*

Lunch

> *300 mg calcium*
>
> *150 mg magnesium*

Supper

> *300 mg calcium*
>
> *150 mg magnesium*
>
> *500 mg vitamin C*
>
> *400 IU vitamin E*

Bedtime

> *300 mg calcium*
>
> *150 mg magnesium*

Chapter 10

The Yoga Healthy Heart Diet Plan

There is no one healthy heart diet profile suitable for everyone. An older person with high cholesterol and a sedentary lifestyle is at much higher risk for heart disease than a younger, more active person with blood fats in the normal range. We recommend you choose one of three different diet plans depending on the following factors and in consultation with your personal physician:

• **Prevention goals:** Are you motivated to change your diet to stay healthy? Follow a moderate diet plan that reduces fat to about 30% of total calories.

• **Risk status:** The more risk factors you have, the lower your total and LDL cholesterol targets should be, and the more aggressive your diet plan.

• **Blood lipid profile:** The higher your blood fats are, especially LDL, total cholesterol, and your total-to-HDL ratio, the more aggressive your diet should be.

• **Difficulty in reducing blood fats:** If you have tried to lower blood cholesterol or fats unsuccessfully before, try a more aggressive diet plan.

• **Artery disease:** Do you know that you already have CHD or perhaps artery blockage in the legs, neck, or elsewhere? I recommend you follow the most aggressive diet plan.

Choosing the Right Diet Plan for You

The idea behind our dietary program is to allow tailoring of your diet to meet your specific needs, from prevention all the way to reversal of existing coronary heart disease (CHD). This chapter outlines three basic diet plans, depending on your goals and risk factors: the "Moderate" plan is for those interested primarily in prevention and is based on current American Heart Association guidelines; it probably will reduce cholesterol about 5%. The "Optimal" plan is for those with two or more risk factors for CHD; it will probably reduce cholesterol about 15%. Finally, the "Aggressive" plan, similar to diets recommended by Dr. Dean Ornish and others, is for those with diagnosed CHD who need to reduce their blood cholesterol considerably; it will probably reduce levels about 30%.

Without doubt, the most important step to take in preventing, halting, or regressing CHD is to reduce total and LDL cholesterol and triglyceride (circulating fat) levels in the blood, and to increase the proportion of HDL cholesterol. To find out which diet plan is best for you, follow these steps:

Step 1. Determine cholesterol level goals. Look at your latest blood cholesterol test results. Find the values for total cholesterol, LDL, HDL, and the "total-to-HDL ratio."

Total cholesterol levels above 160 are associated with increased CHD risk worldwide, so it is important to maintain total cholesterol below 150. LDL cholesterol levels below 130 are generally considered desirable, and the lower the better. Experts currently recommend that LDL be lowered below 100, especially for those with existing CHD, to boost plaque regression.

The concentration of HDL necessary for prevention or regression is likely to change depending on the amount of fat in your diet. As Dr. Ornish has said regarding his very-low-fat diet program, "You have less garbage, so you need fewer garbage men." As I explained in Chapter 1, HDL is responsible for "reverse cholesterol transport," the return of cholesterol from the cells all over the body to the liver for recycling or excretion into the intestines as bile acids. This means that just looking at HDL levels alone — less than 35 too low, above 60 desirable — can be misleading, because levels in the 40s may be entirely adequate if, for example, LDL is 100 or less and total cholesterol is 150 or less.

More important is the proportion of total cholesterol to HDL. Higher levels of total cholesterol need to be balanced by higher levels of HDL to "clean it up"; similarly, if total cholesterol is reduced, lower HDL levels may be fine. A good rule of thumb is for HDL to be one-quarter (25%) or more of total cholesterol — a ratio of 4.0 or lower. For men, a ratio of 5.0 (for women, 4.5) is associated with average risk for CHD. For both sexes, below 3.5 represents a 50% reduction in CHD risk; many experts recommend keeping the ratio at least below 4.0 for a reasonable prevention goal. If, on the other hand, the ratio is larger than 5.0, risk increases: at 9.6 for men (7.1 for women) risk is doubled, and at 24.0 for men (11.0 for women) risk is tripled.

If you currently have no evidence of CHD or other atherosclerotic artery disease, and you have fewer than two risk factors,
your goal is prevention. You should attempt to reduce total cholesterol to below 150 and total cholesterol-to-HDL ratio to 4.0
or below. You should start with the Moderate Diet Plan for six
months, and gradually move to the Optimal or Aggressive Plans
if needed until your blood values are in line with these targets.
In any case, your LDL target is below 130. If you currently have
two or more risk factors but still no evidence of CHD or atherosclerotic artery disease, then you can also start with the Moderate Plan, but your goal should be reducing your LDL to below
115. You should also try to meet the goals described above for
total cholesterol (below 150) and total-to-HDL ratio (below 4.0).

If you have CHD or another atherosclerotic condition affecting arterial blood flow, your goal is regression of blockages. Try
to get LDL below 100. Take your current LDL cholesterol concentration and multiply by 5%, 15%, or 30% to see which plan is
required to lower LDL to 100 or less. For example, if your current LDL value is 135, reducing it by 30% (40.5) would get it below 100, pointing toward the Aggressive Plan. If you cannot
achieve your target in six months of intensive effort, by all means
consult with your health care provider regarding using drug
therapy to supplement — but not replace — your dietary changes
and the other lifestyle changes that are part of our program for
heart health.

Step 2. Determine Your Calorie Level. The number of fat grams
in your selected diet plan is figured as a percentage of total calories. A small, older, sedentary person needs fewer calories (and
thus less dietary fat) than an active younger person and must
restrict fats more to maintain target fat percentages. In general:
smaller people need fewer calories than larger people; women

need fewer calories than men; inactive people need fewer calories than active people. People who need to reduce their weight to a reasonable level need to eat 500 calories fewer per day in order to lose one pound per week. And finally, chronic dieters or athletic people tend to need fewer calories due to a more efficient metabolism. The following calorie guidelines may help you: 1,200 if you are small, female, overweight, sedentary; 1,800 if you are an average-sized woman of moderate activity level or a sedentary man; 2,400 if you are an average-sized man of moderate activity level. See Resources for some books and web sites that can help you refine your calorie needs further for weight loss or maintenance.

Here are some examples of using the formula above for determining the right Diet Plan:

• A small, 50-year-old, sedentary woman, currently with normal lipid levels, slightly overweight, having one close relative with premature CHD (one risk factor), would fall into the prevention category and start the Moderate Diet Plan at the 1,200-calorie level. Goal: Lose weight by reducing calories and increasing activity, and protect heart and arteries by reducing cholesterol intake. Cholesterol levels should decrease to optimum levels.

• A fairly active, normal-weight 48-year-old man, an ex-smoker, with mild high blood pressure (two risk factors) and moderately high blood lipid levels but no symptoms of CHD such as angina would follow the Optimal Diet Plan at the 1,800-2,000 calorie level. Goal: reduce cholesterol and saturated fat consumption so that lipid levels drop to the optimum range. If I were this person, I would also suspect the existence of some mild plaque and fatty lesions and would make these changes to regress any existing artery blockages.

• A large, overweight, 60-year-old, sedentary man with CHD, with a history of chest pain diagnosed as stable angina, would be advised to follow the Aggressive Plan at the 2,400-calorie level. Goal: Lose weight (at least a 10% reduction), gradually become moderately active, and reduce cholesterol and saturated fat intake to the bare minimum. With dedicated effort and comprehensive lifestyle changes, this person has every chance to regress existing artery blockages and virtually eliminate angina symptoms in just a matter of weeks.

Of course, all dietary modifications are meant to be made in association with our other program components of exercise, stress management, and Yoga practices. You will be able to make some increases in caloric intake if you increase the amount of briskly paced exercise you do each day.

Step 3. Refer to the Diet Plan Tables: Fat Allowances. The table on page 208 outlines the fat and cholesterol allowances in each of the Diet Plans. Note for your plan and calorie level the amounts of cholesterol, expressed in milligrams, and the maximum amount of saturated fats, expressed in grams, for daily consumption (the difference between the number for saturated fat and total fat represents the consumption of mono- and polyunsaturated fats). These numbers represent total grams per day. Now, by reading labels and practicing with a few sample menus (see pages 228-231), you can easily guarantee that you stay on the plan. For convenience, we have provided the fat and cholesterol content of some average servings of common foods in the section on how to reduce dietary fats (see pages 221-224).

Daily Calories and Fat Allowances

"Moderate" Plan — 200 mg cholesterol, 30% calories from fat

"Optimal" Plan — 100 mg cholesterol, 20% calories from fat

"Aggressive" Plan — 20 mg cholesterol, 10% calories from fat

		Saturated Fat Allowance (grams)	Total Fat Allowance (grams)
1200 calories	Moderate	8	40
	Optimal	5	27
	Aggressive	4	13
1800 calories	Moderate	12	60
	Optimal	8	40
	Aggressive	6	20
2400 calories	Moderate	17	80
	Optimal	11	53
	Aggressive	9	27

The Food Guide Pyramid

We are basing our suggestions for the healthy heart diet on the USDA Food Guide Pyramid, which suggests how to build your daily diet in terms of servings of different food groups.

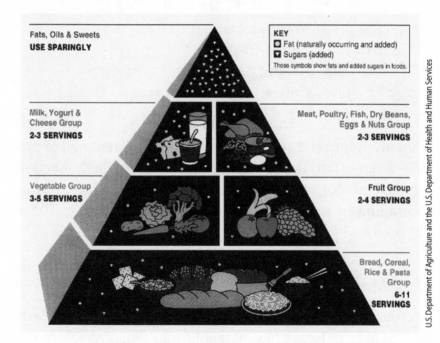

Starting from the lowest, widest level, the food guide pyramid emphasizes carbohydrates, allowing the greatest number of servings for these healthy fuel foods:

Whole Grains:

Whole-grain breads,
cereals (esp. whole oats),
brown rice, and pasta: 6 - 11 servings

Fruits and vegetables:

Deeply colored vegetables: 3 - 5 servings

Colorful or high-fiber fruits: 2 - 4 servings

Protein:

Fat-free dairy
(milk, yogurt, cheese):   2 - 3 servings

Soy products
(reduced-fat or fat-free),
dried beans, peas
and lentils, & nuts: 2 - 3 servings

Fats, oils, and sweets:

Small amount (1-2 teaspoons) of flaxseed oil required to provide essential fatty acids. Use olive or canola sparingly for cooking. Use no (or very little) solid fats, such as lard, butter,
shortening, or stick margarine. Avoid or strictly limit commercial fried foods.

How Many Servings Are Right for You?

If you are older, small in stature, inactive, a chronic dieter, athletic, female, or have a low metabolic rate, you probably have a
really hard time maintaining ideal weight, possibly to the degree that you may even gain weight on a diet that helps your
friends to lose weight! Doubtless, you should lean toward the
low end of the range of servings per day.

On the other hand, bigger (by weight) and younger people, or
those who are moderately to very active, can afford to eat higher
in the range of number of daily servings. Also, men tend to have
higher metabolic rates and can tolerate more servings than
women. Most people will lose a significant amount of weight

when following these diet plans, and a very high percentage suc-cessfully keep it off for years.

What Is a Serving?

Sometimes it can be confusing to figure out what constitutes a serving. Following are a few examples:

- Whole-grain bread – 1 slice
- Ready-to-eat whole-grain cereal – 1 oz (about 1/4 to 1/2 c)
- Cooked whole-grain cereal – 1/2 c
- Cooked brown rice – 1/2 c
- Cooked spaghetti, macaroni, etc. – 1/2 c
- Raw leafy vegetables – 1 c
- Cooked vegetables – 1/2 c
- Vegetable juice – 3/4 c
- Whole fruit (apple, banana, pear, etc.) – 1 med
- Berries, or chopped or cooked fruit – 1/2 c
- Fruit juice – 3/4 c
- Raisins – 1/4 c
- Skim milk – 1 c
- Yogurt, plain, fat-free – 1 c
- Cottage cheese, fat-free – 1/2 c
- Hard cheese, reduced fat or fat-free – 1 1/2 oz
- Dried beans, cooked or canned – 1/2 c
- Nuts – 1 oz
- Tofu – 3 oz
- Vegetarian Canadian bacon and other "fake meats" – 3-4 slices

(Please note: The exact amount of food in an "ounce" can be confusing. Keep yourself honest by investing in an inexpensive food scale available in discount stores.)

How to Reduce Saturated Fats in Your Diet

As I mentioned previously, many studies have shown that most animal fats (from meat and butter) in your diet can increase cholesterol and CHD risk. Here are some suggestions on how to reduce these fats to help yourself lose excess pounds and help your heart at the same time.

Did you know that our taste preference for fatty foods is mostly learned? That means it can be unlearned. Many of my students and I have experienced this in our own lives as we have tried to improve our diets. For instance, many people used to dislike the taste of fat-free milk. By gradually switching to lower fat products, first 2%, then 1%, and finally fat-free, they found that eventually they preferred the taste of the fat-free product and did not miss the totally unnecessary butterfat. Recently some milk producers have improved skim milk simply by adding fat-free milk solids, resulting in even better taste and more fat-free protein and calcium, too; choose these brands whenever you can find them.

Other culturally ingrained habits, such as full-fat ice cream, and sour cream on baked potatoes, can also be changed. (Please don't tell any of my "health food nut" friends, but on a bad day I have been known to use fat-free whipped topping on some fresh berries: it is processed and chemicalized, but has no saturated fat or cholesterol and sometimes it's the only way to get through!) Try fat-free frozen yogurt instead of ice cream, or fat-free yogurt and lemon juice on baked potatoes. My meat-eating friends tell me they have easily re-learned to prefer the taste of the leanest meats, fish, and poultry.

I think it is heartening to find out that when we take pains to break these saturated fat habits, we find that we prefer the taste and texture of foods without the added fat. Take a "saturated fat vacation" for a week or two, and then see what fats you really cannot live without. Add the "must haves" back as sparingly as possible. If you are like most, you can enjoy food and the eating experience just as much with markedly less fat than you are used to, and food flavors will seem to intensify. Here's how to reduce fats in the major food groups of the pyramid:

Whole grains. Try taking the "no-spread pledge." This means eating breads and toast without spreading on the butter or margarine. When eating breakfast in a restaurant, remember to ask for "dry whole wheat toast, please." If at first you can't face toast with no spread at all, try a small amount of no-added-sugar preserves or fat-free cream cheese. There are many packaged cold or hot whole-grain cereals without added sugar available now, though granola is too often a blatant contradiction: widely associated with health, it is often high in both added fat and sugar. Pancakes can be a good choice, especially if you can find some

No-Fat Foolery

Remember that fat-free does not mean calorie-free. Many packaged items have increased sugars and other calorie-dense ingredients in order to compensate for the reduced fat. Read labels, and try to avoid eating packaged foods as much as possible. Especially enjoy the labels on such products as apples, which say "as always, fat-free"!

with fiber, such as buckwheat, and limit the amount of added fat (butter, margarine) and sugar (syrup, jelly) you add.

Do you always put gravy or butter on white rice? Try serving brown rice, which has much more flavor than white, as many Asians do, as a layer under low-fat vegetables or beans, peas, or lentils. Try terrines, loaf-style dishes made with layers of brown rice, vegetables, and beans. Pasta dishes can be low-fat or high-fat items depending on the sauce. Italian-style canned tomato pasta sauces vary from 0% to 50% of calories from fat. Many of the fat-free varieties are quite tasty and are widely available at major supermarkets. Remember, if it is a creamy pasta sauce, it probably is high fat, and saturated to boot. If you really prefer the taste of a creamy sauce, sauté vegetables in a small amount of oil (use a small amount of olive or canola oil, perhaps as a pan spray) and stir fat-free yogurt into the pan after taking it off the heat, to make a low-fat creamy pasta topping. You can also try the more traditional approach of tossing the hot pasta and the sautéed vegetables with crumbled fat-free ricotta cheese. A word about pasta: While technically not whole grain, Italian-style pasta is a slow-release carbohydrate because the wheat is ground instead of milled, yielding a coarser texture that takes longer to digest. Personally, I find the whole grain versions a bit disappointing, and so continue to use the Italian-style ones.

Unfortunately, there is no easy way to reduce the fat in cakes, cookies, and muffins unless you bake them yourself, although low-fat or fat-free products are increasingly available at local supermarkets and bakeries. If you do your own baking, you can substitute nonfat yogurt or applesauce for some or all of the butter or oil in the recipe — and use whole-grain and soy flour for even better nutrition.

How To Cheat

First, don't call it cheating; call it being kind to both your bodies. If you find yourself really hungry between meals, don't give up. Eat an extra whole-grain serving along with a small serving of a protein-rich food; for example, a piece of good whole-grain bread with a glass of fat-free milk. Avoid telling yourself "I've failed, I've blown it, there's no point in continuing," because you have not failed. You have begun a new relationship with your emotional body in a new awareness of its need to be happy. Second, avoid eating fatty foods; even in small portions they won't be as satisfying as a larger portion of whole grains, fruits, or vegetables, with some protein. Remember, complex carbohydrate foods are much less likely to be stored as body fat than the same calories from fatty foods, and they will not elevate your blood fats and cholesterol.

If high-fat bakery items such as cakes, cookies, pie crusts, croissants, and doughnuts are on your list of "must-haves," you'll have to limit them to once a week or less in order to truly benefit from a low-fat diet. Vegetable shortening, while certainly better than butter for baking since it has no cholesterol and about 50% less saturated fat, still contains 3 grams of saturated fat per tablespoon and is high in trans fat content due to hydrogenation.

A good rule of thumb is "Do whatever it takes to avoid bingeing." If you restrict too severely, you may find yourself either saying "I've been really good today so I can have a treat," or following the diet on weekdays and then eating whatever you want on the weekends, or following the diet for three weeks and taking a week off. All these patterns are forms of bingeing based on "Let's make a deal": "I'll give up jelly doughnuts today but you are going to have to give them back to me tonight or next week."

If you find yourself in this type of thought, immediately counteract with the resolution to discover new, healthy enjoyments. Investigate some of the cookbooks recommended in the Resources for treats that will not violate your whole-foods diet. Look upon this way of eating as a way of living, not as though you were saving fatty and sugary goo in your bank account for withdrawal on a rainy day.

Vegetables. Frying vegetables of any kind moves them from the highly recommended list all the way to the "use sparingly" list. The same goes for butter or cheese sauces on vegetables. Flavor your veggies with fresh herbs, lemon juice, and a little salt and pepper, or cook them with onions and garlic. Sauté them quickly in a nonstick pan, with perhaps a teaspoon or two of olive oil, or a quick blast from a canola oil pan spray. Even the large portabello mushrooms can be pan grilled this way. If a butter sauce is on your list of "must haves," try one of the instant natural butter flavor mixes. Vegetables can be sliced and oven roasted, or even grilled; just try not to boil them to death — an old American custom, at least in my childhood home.

Fruits are perhaps the best food for your heart because they are naturally full of potassium, vitamins A and C, and carbohydrates, have a sweet taste, and are usually eaten with no added fat. The only fatty fruit habit that might be a problem is peanut butter on bananas or cream on berries. (I am sure there are many others, but please do not write to tell me about them!) Although peanut butter is high in fat, it is an unsaturated and cholesterol-free fat, so a small amount, depending on your total calorie intake, may be allowed.

Protein: Dairy. At the dairy level of the pyramid, milk and yogurt are readily available in nonfat forms, and some brands of cottage, ricotta, and even Swiss, cream, cheddar, and mozzarella cheeses are available fat-free. We were delighted to discover that even half-and-half can now be purchased in fat-free form, although it still contains over 50% more calories than fortified skim milk.

Protein: Soy Products, Dried Beans, Peas, Lentils, Nuts, and Eggs. Our diet plans are based on a vegetarian structure proven to help the heart, so we suggest that you try to limit your intake of meat as much as possible. Meat, poultry, and fish dishes usually contain high amounts of saturated fat unless special efforts are made to purchase and prepare low-fat versions of typical recipes. Please refer to the fuller discussion of vegetarian and vegan diets later in this chapter, including tips if you feel you must eat meat.

Soy products are increasingly in evidence in major supermarkets, and their low-fat or nonfat varieties are an excellent source of heart healthy protein and isoflavones. Certainly the soy-based "fake meat" wieners, burgers, Canadian bacon, and deli slices are healthier for you than the meats they mimic. Even if you are not a vegetarian, you will benefit from adding some of these foods to your diet; eating a vegetarian "hot dog" or "Canadian bacon" as a snack is a great comfort for hunger pangs. Most people are familiar with soybean curd (tofu), a staple food of Asia; it is a bland, cakelike, high-protein food that can be barbecued, scrambled, sautéed with vegetables, boiled in soup, or baked. When processed with calcium, as it usually is, tofu is a great source of this essential mineral as well as protein. Although nearly 50% of tofu's calories are from fat, the fat is predominantly unsaturated, and at least one major brand has recently introduced an excellent reduced-fat tofu. Refer to Chapter 9, page 175, for delicious ways to increase soy.

Dried beans are traditionally cooked with added fat, and nuts are so high in fat they are even a good commercial source of oil. Nuts are very nutritious, however, containing heart healthy fatty acids and antioxidants. They are low in saturated fat and have no cholesterol, so how much you eat is just a calorie issue.

Perhaps peas and lentils are not so often loaded up with added fats as the other members of the bean group, but even here caution is needed. Split pea and other legume soups traditionally are prepared with added meat fat or fatty broth, and Indian methods of cooking the various legumes (dal) usually call for flavoring with clarified butter (ghee) or fried spices. Eat nontraditional fat-free preparations of peas, beans, and lentils, and limited amounts of nuts. Many of my friends who are trying to eat less meat complain, perhaps rightly so, about the inconvenience of soaking and simmering dried beans and lentils. There is often a slightly shocked expression when I admit to using and enjoying the canned and frozen varieties. One of my favorite quick side dishes is frozen Fordhook lima beans heated with chopped onion, or canned white or kidney beans added to a fresh salad.

Eggs, though low in fat, are the food highest in cholesterol. Try them poached or boiled. Each yolk contains 200-250 mg cholesterol, so allow no more than three to four per week on the Moderate Plan, two on the Optimal Plan, and none on the Aggressive Plan. You can use egg whites, which have no cholesterol and are very high in protein.

How to Read Labels

First, take along reading glasses or a magnifying glass when you go grocery shopping; labels are always printed in tiny type! Along with total calories and other nutritional information, the FDA requires food packagers to list total fat as well as saturated fat; some voluntarily list mono- and polyunsaturated fats as well. Though it may be time-consuming at first, getting into the habit of reading labels on the foods you buy will give you a great deal of knowledge about what you are eating.

Eating in Restaurants

Most restaurants, especially the fast-food establishments, seem to specialize in adding fat to foods in order to enhance the taste. Serving sizes have also grown; in some major chains the amount of food on your plate can easily contain a whole day's requirements of calories. I remember well when a dietician, noting a major food chain's newest big burger, remarked that of course it wasn't too high in fat: just buy one on Monday, cut it into five pieces and eat a piece every day! Fried foods top the list of favorite restaurant foods. If it's fried, it's high in saturated and trans fat, and if it's batter-fried, it's doubly high. That also goes for refried items, cheese sauces, melted cheese, or cream sauce. Almost any whitish dipping sauce is code for mayonnaise, which means high fat and maybe even cholesterol from egg yolks. Always ask for salad dressing on the side, and use as little as you can. I almost always ask for oil and vinegar cruets. You may discover you actually like and prefer the unadorned taste of vegetables.

Salads, bread, and baked potatoes are reasonable choices at most establishments. Deli sandwiches can be improved by replacing mayonnaise with mustard, adding more lettuce, tomato, and onions, using whole-grain bread products, and removing at least half the cheese or meat filling. Chinese food can be a good alternative if you select brothy soups and stir-fried vegetable and bean curd dishes with plain rice. Mexican food should probably be saved for rare special occasions. Fried and refried foods are the order of the day; even avocados are 93% calories from fat. Try to order plain flour tortillas, rice, and beans, and remove extra cheese from items such as tostados, tacos, burritos, and enchiladas. Go easy on the fried corn chip basket offered while you wait.

Feeding Both Your Bodies

If you are cornered by a high-fat burrito, taco, or other food, divide it into three parts. Eat one for your emotional body, one for your physical body, and then fantasize layering the fat from the third part onto your unwilling hips and waist or into your arteries as they protest. If your emotional body fights for more, mark your wrist tape (see page 48) and figure out how to make up the loss to it. This will show you if you are constantly denying your inner emotional body and help you to notice when it rebels. This technique will work with any high-fat or high-sugar foods; you can even divide up all your meals this way just for fun.

Fat and Cholesterol Content of Common Foods

Dairy products & eggs

(Please note that all fat-free dairy has no fat, of course, and only trivial amounts of cholesterol.)

	Sat fat (g)	Mono (g)	Poly (g)	Chol (mg)
Milk, skim, 1 c	0	0	0	4
Milk, 1%, 1 c	2	1	0	10
Milk, 2%, 1 c	3	1	0	18
Cheese, cheddar, 1 1/2 oz	9	4	0	44
Cheese, Swiss, 1 1/2 oz	7	3	0	39
Cheese, mozzarella, whole-milk, 1 1/2 oz	6	3	0	33
Cheese, ricotta, part skim, 1 1/2 oz	2	1	0	14
Cheese, cottage, 2%, 1/2 c	1	1	0	10
Cheese, cream, 2 oz	12	6	1	62
Cheese, cream, fat-free, 2 oz	0	0	0	5
Egg, 1 extra lg	2	2	1	247
Egg white from 1 lg egg	0	0	0	0
Yogurt, plain, 1 c	0	0	0	4
Yogurt, low-fat fruit, 1 c	2	1	0	10
Yogurt, vanilla, 1 c	2	1	0	12
Ice cream, regular vanilla, 1/2 c	4	2	0	29
Ice cream, light, vanilla, 1/2 c	2	1	0	9
Frozen yogurt, vanilla, 1/2 c	2	1	0	1
Ice cream, soft-serve light vanilla, 1/2 c	1	1	0	11
Cottage cheese, fat free, 1/2 c	0	0	0	5

Fats & oils

	Sat fat	Mono	Poly	Chol
Olive oil, 1 T	2	10	1	0
Peanut oil, 1 T	2	6	4	0
Coconut oil, 1 T	12	1	0	0
Canola oil, 1 T	1	8	4	0
Corn oil, 1 T	2	3	8	0
Sunflower oil, 1 T	1	3	9	0
Soybean oil, 1 T	2	3	8	0
Salad dressing, Italian, 1 T	1	2	4	18
Salad dressing, blue cheese, 1 T	2	2	4	3
Salad dressing, French	1	1	3	0
Butter, 1 T	7	3	0	31
Margarine, tub, liquid safflower oil, 1 T	2	1	3	0
Margarine, tub, liquid corn oil, 1 T	0	3	1	0
Margarine, stick, 1 T	2	4	4	0
Vegetable shortening, 1 T	3	6	3	0
Mayonnaise, 1 T	2	3	6	8

Vegetables & legumes

(Vegetarian soy-based "meats" are almost all fat-free. Check labels to make sure.)

	Sat fat	Mono	Poly	Chol
Tofu, 4 oz firm	1	1	3	0
Yves vegetarian Canadian bacon, 4 slices	0	0	0	0

	Sat fat	Mono	Poly	Chol
Tempeh, 4 oz	2	3	4	0
Baked beans, canned, vegetarian, 1 c	0	0	0	0
Vegetarian vegetable soup, canned, 1 c	0	1	1	2

Nuts & seeds

	Sat fat	Mono	Poly	Chol
Almonds, raw, 1 oz	1	9	3	0
Almonds, dry-roasted, 1 oz	1	10	4	0
Peanut butter, chunky, 1 T	2	4	2	0
Sunflower seeds, raw 1 oz	1	3	9	0
Sunflower seeds, dry-roasted, 1 oz	1	3	9	0
English walnuts, raw, 1 oz	2	3	13	0
Macadamia nuts, 1 oz	3	17	0	0
Peanuts, dry-roasted, 1 oz	2	7	4	0

Meat & fish

	Sat fat	Mono	Poly	Chol
Beef, cooked, lean, 3 oz	5	4	1	60
Chicken, cooked, lean, 3 oz	1	2	1	52
Tuna, water-packed, 3 oz	0	0	0	53
Bacon, 2 slices	3	3	1	11
Salmon, baked, 3 oz	6	8	2	15

Grains	(Most commercial and bakery breads are essentially fat-free; here we list only a few grain products that contain some fat.)			
	Sat fat	Mono	Poly	Chol
Ry-Krisp crackers, 2	0	0	1	0
Wheat Thins, 16	1	2	0	0
Triscuits, reduced fat, 7	4	4	1	0
Ritz crackers, 5	1	3	0	0
Quaker 100% Natural cereal, 1/2 c	4	2	1	0

A Healthy Vegetarian Diet

Throughout this book I am emphasizing a healthy, whole-foods vegetarian diet. That is what I have followed for over 45 years, and it is traditionally how serious Yoga students eat, because it is a nonviolent diet that fills your body with positive energy. You do not have to be a vegetarian to practice Yoga, but this type of diet has been well proven to prevent and reverse CHD. It is heartening to me that, after years of vegetarianism being regarded as somewhat "kooky," science has proven that a vegan, vegetarian, or mostly vegetarian diet often prevents or reduces atherosclerotic symptoms.

As a practical matter, it is very difficult to meet low-fat and low-cholesterol criteria with significant portions of meat included. For the Aggressive Diet Plan, it is impossible. The risks of many other chronic conditions, such as arthritis, high blood pressure, diabetes, and even some forms of cancer also can be reduced or even eliminated by a diet rich in whole grains, fruits, and vegetables. It is also true that a healthy vegetarian diet helps you lose weight, because it gives you a greater volume of food to eat, since meat products and processed and refined foods are so calorie-dense. Keep in mind that vegetarian does not necessarily mean low-fat: A grilled cheese sandwich on white bread with French fries may be technically vegetarian, but it is not the kind of food we are talking about in our heart-healthy diet.

A whole-foods diet contains high amounts of cholesterol-lowering fiber. As well, the fiber adds low-calorie bulk to the servings so you are apt to feel satisfied with fewer calories. The fiber content also slows down the absorption of the carbohydrates, lowering the glycemic index of the foods and helping to prevent fat levels rising in carbohydrate-sensitive people. Whole foods also contain many hundreds of beneficial phytochemicals and other natural antioxidants that cannot be obtained any other way.

We recommend a whole-food ovo-lactovegetarian diet, which includes fruits, vegetables, legumes (dried beans and peas), whole grains, seeds, and nuts. The addition of milk and cheese from dairy products, especially the fat-free variety, and egg whites or a few whole eggs (see guidelines above) helps round out the variety of the diet and provide necessary nutrients. Vegetarian diets have a natural advantage over those containing meat as they are typically lower in total fat, saturated fat, and cholesterol.

The Vegan Diet

Vegans, those who eat no animal products of any kind, have the best diet in terms of fat and cholesterol content. A healthy vegan diet is also based almost entirely on whole, as opposed to processed and refined, foods. Nutritionally, the carbohydrate and fat content of a vegan diet is easy: you eat the same whole grains, fruits, and vegetables providing carbohydrates for a nonvegetarian diet. The recommended oils — olive and canola for cooking, with enough flaxseed oil on salads to provide needed essential fatty acids — also work here. You never have to worry about getting too much saturated fat, because there is only a little if you avoid processed foods containing palm, coconut, and cocoa butter fats, and hydrogenated oils. Other oils, legumes, and nuts contain at most one or two grams per serving.

Meeting the recommended protein intake of 15% of total calories is also easy. Soy-based products, including vegetarian "meats," tofu, and tempeh, as well as dried peas, beans, and lentils, are all excellent sources. Soy-milk products are now widely distributed through supermarkets, as are many "fake meat" products, from "bacon" to "chopped hamburger." Rice milk has little protein. Since individual calorie requirements vary quite a bit, an easier way to determine your protein requirements is to multiply your weight by a factor related to your lifestyle. We have provided a table with this calculation for you to refer to (see sidebar, pp. 176-177), and this method usually agrees well with the 15% of total required calories recommended by the USDA.

Many experts have noted over the years that a vegan diet is often deficient in certain vitamins and minerals, and it is true that care is needed to make a vegan diet truly complete. However, it is simple to supplement your diet with the basic multivitamin/mineral supplement as described in the previous chapter. Additionally, some common foods suitable for vegans, such as breads, cereals, and soy/sesame milk, are often fortified with vitamins and minerals. Nutrition experts also counsel in favor of supplementing the essential fatty acid content of a strict diet with foods rich in alpha linolenic acid (ALA), such as flaxseed oil, dark green leafy vegetables, pumpkin seeds, walnuts, and several beans, including soy, kidney, lima, navy, and great northern.

See the Resources section for some recommended whole foods cookbooks that can make switching to a full or partial vegetarian diet much easier.

If You Must Eat Meat

I have known many people over the years who just cannot seem to live without meat. If you feel that you must eat meat, here are some ideas on how to make it less harmful to your heart and arteries:

Fish and poultry generally are lower in saturated fat and cholesterol, especially when prepared without the skin and cooked with no fat or just a little olive oil. Choose the leanest cuts of beef and pork, and grades lower than "prime." It is a good idea to always trim away visible fat and to pour off any fat released by cooking. Better than frying, try baking, broiling, or roasting. Avoid large servings: a standard serving is a three-ounce cooked portion, about the size of the palm of your hand or a deck of cards. Look for low-fat versions of processed sandwich meats, although they are often too high in sodium to be a good choice. Soy versions are much healthier. And perhaps people just do not realize how truly easy it is to substitute for meat servings. One cup cooked beans, peas, or lentils, or three ounces of soybean curd (tofu) or peanut butter, has the same protein as a three-ounce serving of meat.

Sample Menus

To help get you started on your heart-healthy diet, we have put together three sample menus for the 1800-calorie level of the three Diet Plans, showing the fat, protein, and cholesterol content for each day's meals. Add or subtract calories and fat grams if you have chosen either a 1200-calorie or 2400-calorie diet, referring to the chart and instructions on pages 205-208. (See Resources for some excellent books and web sites that can help you easily create your own heart-healthy menus.) Some general rules:

• Choose whole-grain bread, cereals, rolls, brown and wild rice, etc.

• Limit animal protein to about two servings per day of dairy products; in the Aggressive Plan, they must be nonfat choices; the other two plans may include one reduced-fat serving.

• Eggs are permitted occasionally on the Moderate and Optimal Plans, though egg whites would be preferable.

• Avoid processed food as much as possible. If your schedule does not allow much time for cooking, take advantage of commercial low-fat entrees such as those produced by Amy's Kitchen and Healthy Choice.

Moderate Diet Plan

[Approximate values: 1800 daily calories; 51 g (27%) total fat of which 10 g is saturated; 68 g protein; 30 mg cholesterol; grain servings: 7, fruit & vegetable servings: 9, protein servings: 5]

Breakfast   Egg-white omelet with green pepper
and mushrooms

whole-wheat toast with no-sugar-added
preserves

fresh cantaloupe

Lunch   Whole-wheat pita sandwich with tomatoes,
cucumbers, a small amount of feta cheese

apple

pickles

fresh green beans

sliced tomatoes with basil

nonfat fruit-filled cookie

Dinner   Bean burrito with minimal reduced-fat cheese

brown rice

cranberry sauce

green salad

broccoli

sliced orange

Optimal Diet Plan

[Approximate values: 1800 calories; 33 g (17%) total fat of which 7 g is saturated; 72 g protein; 44 mg cholesterol; grain servings: 7, fruit & vegetable servings: 7, protein servings: 5]

Breakfast   Oatmeal, cooked, with small amount chopped walnuts

nonfat milk

strawberries

whole-wheat toast

Lunch   Spicy black bean burger on whole-wheat bun

lettuce, tomatoes, pickles

nonfat vegetable soup

banana

lemon sorbet with raspberries

Dinner   Pasta primavera with small amount of Romano cheese

whole-wheat dinner roll

mixed green salad with beans

Aggressive Diet Plan

[Approximate values: 1800 calories ; 16 g (8%) total fat of which 5 g is saturated; 65 g protein; 24 mg cholesterol; grain servings: 7, fruit & vegetable servings: 9, protein servings: 5]

Breakfast   frozen mixed-grain waffles

small amount maple syrup

blueberries

fat-free cottage cheese

orange juice

Lunch   zucchini lasagna, low-fat

whole-wheat roll

chutney

honeydew melon

minestrone soup

mixed green salad

raspberry sorbet

Dinner   vegetable stew with tofu

brown rice

orange

sliced tomato and cucumber salad

Coronary Heart Disease and Overweight

One of your most important tasks concerning diet and heart disease is achieving and maintaining your ideal weight. As I discussed in Chapter 1, overweight is a major risk factor of CHD, associated with high blood fats and cholesterol, diabetes, and high blood pressure. Losing weight can significantly reduce these conditions and the risk of CHD as well. Unfortunately, the same population most prone to overweight is also most at risk for CHD: older women and men. I can promise you that our whole-foods diet, even though low in fat and cholesterol, can be a lot more interesting than any "fad diet" that you might have tried, and it will help you lose weight and keep it off without starving yourself and causing unhappiness to both your bodies.

Being overweight can hurt your inner body in many ways: Depression, anxiety, and low self-esteem can result from excess weight gain. This makes it essential to find a way to achieve and maintain a normal weight in a healthy way that is also satisfying enough to your inner body that you can continue your new eating and activity habits indefinitely; in other words, to permanently change your lifestyle. Our healthy heart program is all about permanently changing the way you eat, breathe, exercise — even the way you relax!

Achieving and maintaining normal weight is a good way to begin practicing Nonviolence toward yourself. By adding generous amounts of beneficial healthy heart foods and supplements, you have a much better chance of increasing blood flow to the heart, other organs, and muscles, and thus improving your quality of life. I recommend that you do this by balancing diet and physical activity, resulting in greater health and strength while losing weight safely.

Some Tips on How To Lose Weight

1. Use the Wrist Tape Technique. Try to become more aware of how you feel when you eat by trying the Wrist Tape technique (see p. 48 for full instructions). This technique has helped many of my students when they are trying to become more aware of some particular behavior. Place a piece of nonirritating tape (first-aid adhesive tape, painter's masking tape, or a simple Band-Aid works well) on your wrist every day for one week. Whenever you eat something, write "F" on the tape if you are eating because you need fuel, "B" if you are eating because you are lonely, depressed or bored, or "S" if you are stressed. At the end of the week, add up the three categories to show you how your mood affects how you eat. If you often eat when bored or stressed, that should indicate to you that it is important to find some substitute activities to nourish and care for your emotional needs; otherwise, it will be much harder to lose weight. Make a list of other things to do instead of eating and post it where it will do the most good: on the fridge!

2. Follow the old saying, "Eat breakfast like a king, lunch like a prince, and supper like a pauper." It really does make a difference when you eat, because calories consumed when you are inactive — which for most people is at the end of the day — are more likely to be stored as fat. Fuel up before the most active part of your day and you will also be less likely to "diet" all day and "blow it" at night.

3. Learn your caloric needs for simply maintaining your current weight (see Resources for some good books and other help).

Subtract 500 calories daily to lose a pound per week. The calories saved can also come from increased aerobic activity: you can figure about 300 calories are burned for each hour of moderately paced exercise such as brisk walking (see Chapter 8).

Important Note: I do not recommend eating fewer than 1,200 calories per day without strict physician supervision, because fasting and extremely low-calorie diets have severe effects on your body's metabolism. If you wish to lose excess weight, you may need to boost your activity level so that you can lose weight on 1,200 calories. Remember that strengthening, aerobic, and Yoga exercises are all good ways to restore activity levels to strengthen your heart. These activities also increase your muscle mass and metabolic rate, which helps to keep weight off for the long term. For each 30 minutes of brisk activity each day, you can add back 135 calories (180 for men). Additional exercise is the best solution also for smaller people who hit the 1,200-calories limit, because they can increase weight loss goals without reducing calories to dangerous levels.

4. Eat meals sitting down, and pace your eating, because it takes at least 20 minutes for the food to enter your bloodstream, sending a signal to your brain that you've had enough. Eat slowly and enjoy your meal. It is often a good idea to start with a low-calorie salad or a broth-type soup to make the meal last longer and fill you up sooner.

5. Do not try to deprive yourself of your favorite foods. The most likely outcome of dieting in my experience is "reward bingeing," where we say to ourselves, "I've been good all day, now I deserve that jelly doughnut (or a double date — you know, the one with Ben and Jerry!"). Enjoy a small portion of your favorite food once a week: look forward to it, enjoy it, savor each yummy, greasy creamy bite! — and then move on.

6. Use the Yoga Fantasy techniques (see Chapter 7) to build a picture of yourself as you want to be: thinner, lighter, filled with health, free from pain, and so on. Start your day by filling your mind with positive visions of yourself to counteract feelings of failure and frustration that are actually violent toward yourself and lead to the urge to eat the wrong foods.

7. Find an exercise program you can follow. Despite what the popular magazines try to tell you, there is no magic pill or instant-success system for either curing CHD or losing weight. There is no getting around the simple fact that to lose weight you must eat fewer calories than you burn up in physical activity. This of course becomes more difficult when angina pain discourages calorie-burning exercise. The same exercises that help strengthen the heart are also good for calorie burning. It is essential to increase your activity level by following the routines outlined in this book; a nutritious diet cannot provide enough essential nutrients and still be low enough in calories for your body to burn fat if you are inactive.

When you are inactive, your muscles start wasting away, and your percentage of body fat soars. Muscles burn many more calories than fat, so with less muscle mass, you would have to restrict your calorie intake even more just to maintain weight, much less lose extra pounds. It is also important to remember that metabolism naturally slows down with age, so a constant activity level is necessary to counteract these additional effects. The Yoga exercises presented in Chapter 4 help to maintain the most efficient metabolism; they are easy enough that they can be done every day, and many can be adapted for practice in a chair or even in bed, so the benefits can continue despite injury, illness, or age.

8. Cut out the junk food. The easiest and healthiest way to lose weight consistently, besides exercising regularly, is to reduce your intake of the nonessential calories from the "calorie-dense" foods: mostly processed or artificial foods high in fat, salt, and/ or simple sugar but low in nutrients. A recent nutrition report showed that about one-third of Americans consume nearly half of their daily calories from such "junk" foods. When you throw out the junk, you will be left with plenty of nutritious food to eat that not only build health, but also satisfy your hunger.

In this and the previous chapter, I have presented a detailed outline of how to change your eating habits so that you can supply the raw materials to protect and rebuild your arteries. The Yogic approach to CHD and diet is a lifestyle change that will help you all your life. When you eat well without abusing your physical body with food, you will feel better, have more energy to exercise and engage in activities that you love, and take the biggest step you can toward preventing or regressing heart disease.

Resources

Heart Disease — General

Dr. Dean Ornish's Program for Reversing Heart Disease (Ivy Books/ Ballantine, 1990/1996)

Stress, Diet and Your Heart, by Dr. Dean Ornish (New American Library, 1991)

Nutrition Information / Diet Plans / Calorie Counts

Nancy Clark's Sports Nutrition Guidebook, 2nd ed., by Nancy Clark (Champaign, IL: Human Kinetics, 1996).

The Nutrition Doctor's A-to-Z Food Counter, by Dr. Ed Blonz (New York: Penguin, 1999).

Prevention Magazine's Nutrition Advisor, by Mark Bricklin (Emmaus, PA: Rodale Press, 1993).

"Nutrition Action" (newsletter of the Center for Science in the Public Interest, 1875 Connecticut Ave., NW, #300, Washington, DC 20009-5729). Up-to-date information for consumers about food safety, nutrition research, healthy eating suggestions, and so on.

Whole Foods / Vegetarian Cookbooks

(Many of these titles feature a nutrient analysis for each recipe.)

Everyday Cooking with Dr. Dean Ornish (Harper Collins, 1997)

Cooking with the Right Side of the Brain, by Vicki Rae Chelf (Avery, 1991)

Eat More, Weight Less, by Dr. Dean Ornish (HarperPernennial, 1993)

Moosewood Low-fat Favorites, by the Moosewood Collective (Clarkson Potter, 1996)

Vegetarian Times Low-Fat and Fast (MacMillan, 1997)

1001 Low-Fat Vegetarian Recipes, by Sue Spitler (2nd ed) (Surrey Books, 2000)

Becoming Vegetarian: The Complete Guide to Adopting a Vegetarian Diet, by Vesanto Melina, Brenda Davis, and Victoria Harrison (Summertown, TN: The Book Publishing Co., 1995)

Helpful Websites

Following are a few helpful websites available as of the publication of this book. In addition to basic information about healthy weight management, many of these sites offer interactive tools such as individual diet planners and food analysis, a chance to ask experts questions about dieting and nutrition, support chat rooms, and other features. (Because the content of the World Wide Web changes constantly, use search engines to find a current list of helpful sites.)

americanheart.org
  (American Heart Association)
cyberdiet.com ("healthy heart")
eatright.org
  (American Dietetic Association, search "heart")
fatfree.com
heartinfo.org
ificinfo.health.org
intelihealth.com ("heart")
prevention.com (heart health quiz)
vegsource.com
webmd.com ("Dean Ornish, MD lifetsyle")

Diet and Weight Loss Professionals

Registered Dieticians

For individualized advice about a weight loss or heart-healthy diet, we recommend consulting a registered dietician (RD). These health professionals have fulfilled specific educational requirements, have passed a registration exam, and are a recognized member of the nation's largest organization of nutrition professionals, The American Dietetic Association. Contact them for a referral to a professional in your area.

American Dietetic Association
216 W. Jackson Blvd.
Chicago, IL 60606-6995
Tel: 312-899-0040 x4750
Fax: 312-899-4739
website: www.eatright.org

800-366-1655 (toll-free) for recorded messages about current nutrition topics and to get a referral to a registered dietician in your local area.

900-225-5267 for individualized answers to your questions from a registered dietician. Charges: $1.95 first minute, $.95 each additional minute, average call four minutes.

Weight Loss Physicians

Call local area hospitals (some have special weight-loss clinics) or look for advertisements in your Yellow Pages or newspaper Health section.

Contact the American Society of Bariatric Physicians. This is a voluntary organization; physicians with the best credentials will also be Diplomates of the American Board of Bariatric Medicine; they will have passed both on on-site, peer-reviewed Patient Care Review and an extensive written and oral board exam.

> American Society of Bariatric Physicians
> 5600 S. Quebec St. #109A
> Englewood, CO 80111

(303) 779-4833 to obtain a list of referrals by mail or fax (CO residents in area code 303 call 770-2526, ext. 10); or visit their website: www.asbp.org

Physician referrals are also available online at www.obesity-news.com

Books on Walking, Swimming, and Cycling

Walking Medicine, by Gary Yanker (McGraw-Hill, 1992)

Walk Aerobics, by Les Snowdon (Overlook Press, 1995)

WALKFIT for a Better Body, by Kathy Smith (Warner Books, 1994)

Fitness Cycling, by Chris Carmichael and Edmund R. Burke (Human Kinetics, 1994)

Power Pacing for Indoor Cycling, by Kristopher Kory and Thomas Seabourne (Human Kinetics, 1999)

Cycling Past 50, by Joe Friel (Human Kinetics, 1998)

All-American Aquatic Handbook, by Jane Katz (Allyn & Bacon, 1996)

Swimming for Total Fitness, by Jane Katz (Main Street Books, rev. ed. 1993)

Complete Book of Swimming, by Dr. Phillip Whitten (Random House, 1994)

Healing Moves: how to cure, relieve, and prevent common ailments with exercise, by Carol Krucoff and Mitchell Krucoff (Harmony Books, 2000)

Resources from the American Yoga Association

Further information on Yoga is available from the American Yoga Association. To obtain free information about Yoga, including a complete catalog and guidelines for choosing a qualified teacher, visit our website, or send a self-addressed envelope stamped with postage for two ounces to the following address:

American Yoga Association
P.O. Box 19986
Sarasota, FL 34276

If you have a specific question about Yoga and would like a personal reply, write to the address above, or contact us by telephone, fax, or E-mail:

Telephone (941) 927-4977
Fax: (941) 921-9844
E-mail: info@americanyogaassociation.org
Website: www.americanyogaassociation.org

We offer classes in the Cleveland, Ohio, area. For more information, write or call:

American Yoga Association
P.O. Box 18105
Cleveland Hts, OH 44106
Telephone (216) 556-1313

Books

The American Yoga Association Beginner's Manual (Simon & Schuster, 1987). Complete instructions for over 90 Yoga exercises and breathing techniques; three 10-week curriculum outlines, and chapters on nutrition, philosophy, stress management, nutrition, pregnancy, and more.

The American Yoga Association's New Yoga Challenge (NTC/Contemporary, 1997). Routines for Energy, Strength, Flexibility, Focus, and Stability offer more vigorous Yoga workouts for body and mind. The last chapter, "The Powerful Individual," teaches you how to design your own routine.

The American Yoga Association Wellness Book (Kensington, 1996). A basic routine to maintain health and well-being, plus chapters on how Yoga can specifically help with arthritis, heart disease, back pain, PMS & menopause, weight management, insomnia, headaches, and eight other health conditions.

The American Yoga Association's Yoga for Sports (NTC/Contemporary Books, 2000). A comprehensive book for every athlete, including techniques for bringing the physical and emotional bodies together to attain peak performance. Includes a core routine of exercise, breathing, and meditation, plus specific exercise routines for dozens of individual sports, team sports, and coaches.

Arthritis: An American Yoga Association Wellness Guide (Kensington Books, 2001). A complete program for management of osteo- and rheumatoid arthritis in six parts: Yoga exercise, breathing, and meditation, combined with fantasy techniques, a special walking program, diet and nutrition recommendations, and advice on alternative therapies.

Conversations with Swami Lakshmanjoo, Volume I: Aspects of Kashmir Shaivism (American Yoga Association, 1995). Edited transcripts of Alice Christensen's interviews with Swami Lakshmanjoo, talking about his childhood and early years in Yoga, plus some basic concepts in the philosophy of Kashmir Shaivism.

Conversations with Swami Lakshmanjoo, Volume II: The Yamas and Niyamas of Patanjali (American Yoga Association, 1998).

Edited transcripts of Alice Christensen's dialogues with Swami Lakshmanjoo about these essential ethical guidelines in Yoga.

Easy Does It Yoga (Fireside/Simon & Schuster, 1999). For those with physical limitations, this book includes instruction in specially adapted Yoga exercises that can be done in a chair or in bed, breathing techniques, and meditation.

The Easy Does It Yoga Trainer's Guide (Kendall-Hunt, 1995). A complete manual for how to begin teaching the Easy Does It Yoga program to adults with physical limitations due to age, convalescence, substance abuse, injury, or obesity. Excellent for health professionals, activities directors, physical therapists, home health aides, and others who work with the elderly or in rehabilitative services.

The Light of Yoga (American Yoga Association, 1997). A chronicle of the unusual circumstances that catapulted Alice Christensen into Yoga practice in the early 1950s, including the teachers and experiences that shaped her first years of study.

Meditation (American Yoga Association, 1994). A collection of excerpts from lectures and classes on the subject of meditation, including a section of questions and answers from students.

20-Minute Yoga Workouts (Ballantine, 1995). Brief routines that anyone can fit into the busiest schedule. Includes chapters on women's issues, including pregnancy, toning and shaping, the "20-minute challenge," and workouts to do when you're away from home.

Reflections of Love (American Yoga Association, 1994). A collection of excerpts from Alice Christensen's lectures and classes on the subject of love.

Weight Management: An American Yoga Association Wellness Guide (Kensington Publishing, 2001). A complete program for weight management in six parts: Yoga exercise, breathing, and meditation, combined with fantasy techniques, a special walking program, and a healthy and enjoyable diet plan.

Yoga of the Heart: Ten Ethical Principles for Gaining Limitless Growth, Confidence, and Achievement (Daybreak/Rodale Books, 1998). A clear, direct presentation of ten essential ethics — Nonviolence, Truthfulness, Nonstealing, Celibacy, Nonhoarding, Purity, Contentment, Tolerance, Study, and Remembrance — that help a person realize the power and support of joining the physical and spiritual bodies. Each chapter includes suggestions for how to start practicing, common pitfalls along the way, and many examples from students' experiences and mythology to illustrate the journey.

Audiotapes

Complete Relaxation and Meditation with Alice Christensen. A two-tape audiocassette program that features three guided meditation sessions of varying lengths, including instruction in a seated posture, plus a discussion of meditation experiences.

The "I Love You" Meditation Technique. This technique begins with the experience of a more conscious connection with the breath through love. It then extends this feeling throughout the body and mind in relaxation and meditation. This tape teaches you the beauty of loving yourself and it removes unseen fear.

Videotapes

Basic Yoga. A complete introduction to Yoga that includes exercise, breathing, and relaxation and meditation techniques. Provides detailed instruction in all the techniques including variations for more or less flexibility, plus a special limbering routine and back-strengthening exercises. Features a 30-minute daily routine demonstrated in the setting of a Yoga class.

Conversations with Swami Lakshmanjoo. A set of three videotapes in which Alice Christensen introduces Swami Lakshmanjoo and talks with him about his background, the philosophy of Kashmir Shaivism, and other topics in Yoga. (Some material corresponds to the book *Aspects of Kashmir Shaivism,* described above.)

The Yamas and Niyamas: A Videotape Study Program. A complete set of 25 videotapes of Alice Christensen's comprehensive lectures on the ethical guidelines that form the cornerstone of Yoga philosophy and practice.

The Hero in Yoga: A Videotape Study Program. A series of 24 videotaped lectures by Alice Christensen on Joseph Campbell's landmark text *The Hero With a Thousand Faces*, showing how the adventure of the hero, represented in mythologies all over the globe, parallels the Yoga student's search for self-actualization.

How to Choose a Qualified Yoga Teacher

So far, no national or international certification program for Yoga teachers exists, and it is unlikely that it will, because of the traditional nature of Yoga instruction. For many thousands of years, Yoga was transmitted from teacher to student on a one-to-one basis; only comparatively recently has Yoga been offered in a group class format. Advanced practice of Yoga still is best undertaken on a one-to-one basis, if you are lucky enough to find a competent teacher who is willing to teach you. In my opinion, teaching Yoga should not be viewed as a hobby or a sideline undertaken by someone who reads a couple of books and decides to become a Yoga teacher; he or she must be under the constant supervision of his or her personal Yoga teacher. This relationship between teacher and student is taken very seriously by both parties and is never entered into lightly.

People are constantly asking us to recommend teachers in their area. Because of my belief in the strict training required for the teaching of Yoga, I have made it a policy never to recommend a teacher unless I have trained the person. I cannot take responsibility for other people's teaching. This does not mean that there are no competent teachers available; you may just have to search a little harder. If you are not sure where to start looking, inquire about adult education programs at local schools, look for flyers posted in local health food stores and bookstores or notices in community papers, and inquire at dance and massage studios.

In the following paragraphs, I have outlined what I believe are the minimum requirements for a competent teacher of Yoga.

1. Daily practice of Yoga exercise, breathing, and meditation. No one can make progress in Yoga without a serious commitment to daily practice. A teacher must have this support in order to build the solid foundation of experience that is required before he or she can show others how to achieve that experience; daily practice is also needed to maintain the strength and health necessary for the extra demands of teaching.

2. Regular contact with a teacher. No teacher can work effectively in a vacuum, and no one becomes so advanced that he or she does not need the guidance and support of his or her own teacher.

3. Study of the important Yoga texts. Study is one of the five observances that are part of the essential eight "limbs" of Yoga practice (see #4, below). A teacher needs to have an intensive background of study that includes Patanjali's *Yoga Sutras*, the *Hatha Yoga Pradipika*, the *Bhagavad Gita*, and all world philosophies, at the very least.

4. Ethical behavior. The five *yamas* (meaning "restraints": nonviolence, truthfulness, nonstealing, periods of celibacy, nonhoarding) and the five *niyamas* (meaning "observances": purity, contentment, tolerance, study, remembrance) are the first two limbs in Patanjali's system of classical Yoga (called "Ashtanga Yoga"). The remaining six limbs are 1) physical exercises (*asana*), 2) breathing techniques (*pranayama*), 3) withdrawal of the mind from the senses (*pratyahara*), 4) concentration, defined as selective and voluntary dishabituation (*dharana*), 5) meditation (*dhyana*), and 6) absorption, or ultimate union with the self (*samadhi*). My teacher Lakshmanjoo once said that, like a child developing in the womb whose limbs grow all at once, rather than one by one, these eight limbs must be developed simultaneously.

The ethical guidelines of the yamas and niyamas are a part of Yoga practice not for moralistic reasons but because they support and protect the student during the unfolding of personal experience in meditation. A teacher needs this support and protection for the same reasons as well as to help reduce the interference of personal ego in the teaching process.

An ethical Yoga teacher conducts classes in a responsible, safe, and aware manner; organizes classes that are not too large for each student to receive individual attention; and never pushes students beyond their limitations. Sexual involvement with students is absolutely prohibited.

5. A healthy vegetarian diet. Although you do not need to be a vegetarian to practice Yoga, a Yoga teacher must conform to different standards. Someone who is taking responsibility for teaching others how to use Yoga meditation techniques must have the steadiness and nonviolent attitude that can only be attained through a vegetarian diet. It goes without saying that a teacher should not smoke or use drugs (other than prescription medication) or misuse alcohol.

6. Training in basic anatomy and the effects of Yoga techniques. A teacher must be able to vary the techniques according to each student's ability and know how to advise students with common medical conditions such as hypertension, arthritis, and back problems. I also believe that a teacher should be able to recognize when a student needs professional psychological counseling and be familiar with community services to which to refer the student.

7. Ability to separate Yoga from religion. I have seen many poor-quality instructors take on the trappings and robes of Hinduism or some other religion to give themselves an authority through packaging rather than through the authenticity of their own Yoga practice. This practice severely misrepresents Yoga. Yoga is not a religion; it predates Hinduism — as well as all known religious practices — and its techniques have been used throughout the world. Yoga is a system of nonreligious, transcultural techniques that can develop greater self-knowledge and awareness. Unlike a religion, Yoga does not require adherence to certain creeds or beliefs, nor does it require obeisance to any particular prophet or god. Yoga is not ritualistic, nor is it occult. The texts of Yoga are not scriptures but rather handbooks or guidelines of how to use the techniques safely and what kinds of experiences might be possible. Everyone has a right to their personal religious beliefs, but a teacher must never impose his or her personal beliefs on students in a Yoga class.

About the American Yoga Association

The American Yoga Association teaches a comprehensive and balanced program of Yoga that includes the Hatha Yoga exercises and breathing techniques as well as meditation. Rather than stressing physical culture for its own sake, our core curriculum acknowledges the deeper possibilities of Yoga by teaching meditation and by encouraging the inner-directed awareness that eventually leads to greater self-knowledge. This reliance on individual experience and feeling is a central theme in the science of Yoga, and it underlies the philosophical system of Kashmir Shaivism which supports our line of teaching. Our goal is to offer the highest quality Yoga instruction possible. There are two American Yoga Association Centers in the United States.

About the Author

Alice Christensen stands out as a Yoga teacher with the rare ability to make the often-complex ideas and techniques of Yoga accessible to our Western outlook and lifestyle. She established the American Yoga Association in 1968, the first nonprofit organization in the United States dedicated to education in Yoga.

She has consistently presented Yoga in a clear, classical manner for over forty years. She presents Yoga without dogma or prescription, as a potent avenue for individual inquiry. She has designed programs of Yoga that can be used to enhance any lifestyle. Whether the goal is to maintain health or to explore the nature of the self, her programs can be used to achieve a wide range of goals.

Index